Getting Your PhD
A Practical Insider's Guide

Getting Your PhD
A Practical Insider's Guide

Harriet Churchill and **Teela Sanders**

Office of Academic Programs
Nazarene Theological Seminary
1700 East Meyer Blvd.
Kansas City, MO 64131-1246

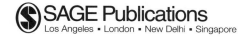

SAGE Publications
Los Angeles · London · New Delhi · Singapore

SAGE Publications Ltd
1 Oliver's Yard
55 City Road
London EC1Y 1SP

SAGE Publications Inc.
2455 Teller Road
Thousand Oaks, California 91320

SAGE Publications India Pvt Ltd
B 1/I 1 Mohan Cooperative Industrial Area
Mathura Road, Post Bag 7
New Delhi 110 044

SAGE Publications Asia-Pacific Pte Ltd
33 Pekin Street #02-01
Far East Square
Singapore 048763

Library of Congress Control Number 2006938309

British Library Cataloguing in Publication data

A catalogue record for this book is available from the British Library

ISBN 978-1-4129-1993-7
ISBN 978-1-4129-1994-4 (pbk)

Typeset by C&M Digital (P) Ltd., Chennai, India
Printed in Great Britain by The Cromwell Press Ltd, Trowbridge, Wiltshire
Printed on paper from sustainable resources

Contents

Contents   vii

Acknowledgements

This book would not have been possible without the twenty-seven contributors who so willingly shared their experiences. We thank all of them for their thoughtful reflection and commitment to the project. Harriet would like to thank those who undertook the PhD journey with her, namely Ruth, Ali and Erica. Teela would like to acknowledge the role of her current PhD students who have provided renewed enthusiasm for passing on knowledge and building a research community. Thanks must go to Patrick Brindle at Sage Publications for his faith in our ideas, his thoroughness and his patience.

Contributors

Bill Armer undertook an 'access' course at the age of 42 in Scarborough, going on to study at Leeds University for a BA in Social Policy. On graduating he took a 'real world' job for a year before returning to Leeds to study for an MA in Disability Studies, and subsequently embarked upon PhD research into the social policy implications of eugenic ideology during the twentieth century. He is the author of 'In Search of a Social Model of Disability: Marxism, normality and culture' (which appeared as a chapter in Barnes, C. and Mercer, G. (2004) *Implementing the Social Model of Disability: Theory and Research*. Leeds: The Disability Press).

JK Tina Basi is among the first graduates from the PhD programme in Gender Studies at the Centre for Interdisciplinary Gender Studies (CIGS), University of Leeds. Her thesis, titled *Globalization and Transnational Indian Call Centres: Constructing Women's Identities*, is soon to be published. Born in Nottingham, raised in Canada and having worked abroad and travelled extensively, her research interests involve feminist theory, globalisation, race and ethnicity, diaspora studies, technology and transnational subjectivities. As an Indian feminist and artist she has also produced and performed in the premier UK charity production of the *Vagina Monologues*, and written numerous short stories, screenplays, and stage plays. She currently works at Intel Ireland in the Digital Health Group on a number of research projects including the Global Ageing Experience, for which she is conducting ethnographic, qualitative research on elderly people around the world.

Ruth Bartlett is a lecturer in dementia studies at the University of Bradford. She is co-ordinator for the BSc in Dementia Studies and Older People's Health in Mind Peer Educator Course, she also teaches on the MSc in Dementia Studies. She has a professional background in mental health nursing, which involved working with people with dementia in a wide range of clinical and social care settings. Ruth graduated from Oxford Brookes University in 2004 with a PhD in sociology. Her doctorate explored meanings of social exclusion in relation to older people with dementia in care homes. Current research interests include the civic participation of people with dementia and cultural conceptions of citizenship.

Marta Bolognani holds a lecturership in Anthropology at the Lahore University of Management Sciences, Pakistan. While being unemployed she was pursuing a career as a professional Bollywood dancer, but academia won her over. At the moment she is turning her doctoral research in the cultural aspects of crime and crime prevention in the Pakistani community for Bradford into a book. She is the convenor of the Pakistan Workshop in the Lake District. Her main interests are British Pakistanis' identity, Muslims' identity, transnationalism and anthropological research methods.

Jonny Burnett is currently finishing a PhD at the Centre for Criminal Justice Studies, University of Leeds. His research interests include contemporary immigration and asylum policy, 'anti-terrorism' policies, policing, and community cohesion. He has written in a variety of publications – 'academic' and otherwise – around these concerns, including *Race and Class*, *Journal for Crime, Conflict and the Media*, *Campaign Against Racism and Fascism*, and *Red Pepper*.

Joseph Burridge spent seven and a half years in the School of Sociology and Social Policy at the University of Nottingham, first as a sociology undergraduate and then as a postgraduate at both masters and PhD level. He wrote his masters thesis on the then failed process of repealing Section 28, and then received an ESRC grant to fund his PhD research into the 'discursive difficulty' observable in social conflicts, and in the build-up to the invasion of Iraq in 2003 specifically. He is currently a Research Associate on the *Changing Families, Changing Food* programme at the University of Sheffield.

Harriet Churchill is a Lecturer in Social and Public Policy (University of Manchester) and has also worked as a Research Fellow (University of Leeds) and an Associate Lecturer (The Open University). Harriet's research interests span research methods, welfare reform, contemporary family lives and theories that explore relationships between identity formation, agency and social structures. Harriet completed her PhD on *Lone Motherhood: Identity and Agency in Context* in 2004 at Oxford Brookes University and has publications on New Labour's family policy, the development of children's services, lone mothers' accounts of parenting and the PhD experience.

Sharon Elley is currently studying for her doctorate at the University of Leeds. She is a part-time lecturer in sociology and has been a youth worker for six years. Her research interests centre on young people's issues, supporting them and acknowledging their views within society, particularly within formal and informal education. Her PhD research focuses upon young people's views of sex and relationship education, sexuality and close, intimate relationships in general.

Sallyann Halliday is a Research Fellow at the Policy Research Institute, Leeds Metropolitan University and a part-time PhD student in the School of Sociology and Social Policy at the University of Leeds. Her main areas of research interest are worklessness, social inclusion and the research process. Her work has recently included being a member of the 'Worklessness' team as part of the national evaluation of 'New Deal for Communities' and lead researcher for the 'Gorbals' in Glasgow as part of the national evaluation of 'Working Neighbourhood Pilots'. Her PhD research is exploring the world of contract research, focusing on negotiated knowledge production and occupational culture.

Richard Heslop is researching for a Doctorate in Education at the University of Leeds and his main research interest lies in the areas of police training and police culture. When he started his doctorate Richard was a part-time student and full-time police officer, though he now realises that this relationship has become the other way round! He has a BSc in social science from the Open University, an MA in politics from the University of Leeds and a PGCE from Huddersfield.

Yousaf Ibrahim is a senior lecturer in Sociology at Trinity and All Saints College, Leeds. He is currently completing his doctorate in the School of Sociology and Social Policy at the University of Leeds. His research is focused on the international protests against new-liberal globalisation and the conflicts between different organisation and participants in the anti-capitalist movement.

Rebecca Mallett is a disabled researcher who has recently submitted her PhD thesis. Her research focuses around contemporary intersections between cultural theory and disability studies. She is also the coordinator for the Postgraduate/Doctoral Disability Research Forum (Centre of Applied Disability Studies, University of Sheffield) which, in part, involves organising workshops on inclusive practices for disability-related research.

Claire Maxwell is a research officer at the Thomas Coram Research Unit, Institute of Education, University of London. Her area of expertise is young people's experiences of sexual and intimate relationships, with a specific focus on young women and agency. Prior to receiving her PhD (2005) from the University of London, she studied for her MA, MSc and Diploma of Social Work at the University of Oxford. Claire's background has been in social work, youth policy development and teaching on the Open University's 'Working with Young People' course. Recent publications have appeared in *Journal of Youth Studies* and *Journal of Adolescence*.

Doug Morrison is studying for a doctorate at the Department of Law, University of Leeds. The focus of his research concentrates on three core areas: bioethical issues surrounding clinical and research practice and the impact of both professional guidance and the law, all set against the background of events at both Alder Hey Children's Hospital and Bristol Royal Infirmary and the non-consensual retention of organs and tissues. The impetus for these interests can be traced to both his previous career in the NHS, where he worked in a variety of clinical and research settings, as well his completion of the LLB at the University of Leeds.

Eve Parsons is a UKCP registered psychotherapist working full time in the student counselling service at Nottingham Trent University. She works with individuals and groups, including support groups for postgraduate students.

John Michael Roberts is a lecturer in sociology and communications at Brunel University. He received his PhD in 2000 from Cardiff University. Research interests can be seen in his publications, which include *The Aesthetics of Free Speech* (Palgrave, 2003), *Realism, Philosophy and Social Science* (co-authored, Palgrave, 2006), *After Habermas: New Perspectives on the Public Sphere* (co-edited, Blackwell, 2004), *Realism, Discourse and Deconstruction* (co-edited, Routledge, 2004) and *Critical Realism and Marxism* (co-edited, Routledge 2002). He is currently working on a new book that explores the different forms of free speech in the global world today.

Christine Rogers is a Lecturer in Education in the School of Criminology, Education, Sociology and Social Work at Keele University. She completed her PhD, titled *A Sociology of Parenting Children Identified with Special Educational Needs: The Private and Public Spaces Parents Inhabit*, at the University of Essex and then spent a year as an ESRC postdoctoral research fellow in the Centre for Family Research, University of Cambridge. Christine has published in *Auto/Biography* and *British Journal of Sociology of Education*. She has also written (with Helen Lucey) on the power relationship between the supervisor and research student in a book *Power, Knowledge and the Academy: Exploring the Institutional and Personal Dynamics of Feminist Research*, commissioned by Palgrave. Christine is now researching sexual identity and young adults with learning impairments and not coincidently, has a teenage daughter with learning impairments.

Teela Sanders is a Senior Lecturer in Sociology of Crime and Deviance in the School of Sociology and Social Policy, University of Leeds. Her current research interests are in the areas of gender, regulating behaviours and deviance and she has conducted extensive research in the sex industry. She has journal articles in, amongst others, *Sociology, British Journal of Sociology, Gender, Work and Organization, Urban Studies*, and *Feminist Criminology*. Teela has published the books *Sex Work: A Risky Business* (Willan, 2005) and more recently *Paying for Pleasure: Men Who Buy Sex* (Willan, 2007).

Nicola Scott is a doctoral candidate in the Department of Government, International Politics and Philosophy, University of Manchester. Her research looks at the international political economy of North–South, 'private–public' partnerships to foster capacity building in crop biotechnology within developing countries.

Sonali Shah has just completed a three-year postdoctorate at the University of Nottingham, on a project funded by the European Social Fund: 'Future Selves: Career Choices of Young Disabled People'. The study explores the choices of disabled young people, and the structures and policies in the education system, through innovative drama techniques, qualitative interviews with young people and relevant education professionals. It also uses her experience as a young disabled researcher to develop understanding of the perspective of young disabled people, which is often ignored.

Melanie Shearn is currently a full-time PhD student at the University of Leeds. Her research is on fathers, choice-making and work–life balance issues and policies, and is funded by the ESRC. She has worked in a variety of jobs in both the UK and South Africa.

Martin Smith is currently employed as a Senior Intelligence Analyst by Bedfordshire Police, where he analyses patterns and trends in local criminality, as well as profiling offenders and crime problems. Prior to leaving academia, Martin was employed by the University of Oxford for two years as a Research Officer in Demography at the Department of Social Policy and Social Work. He studied for a PhD in Geography at the University of Oxford from 1997–2001, looking at the life-chances and aspirations of young people of Bangladeshi origin living in east London. This followed completion of his first degree in Geography at Lancaster University, from where he graduated in 1996.

David Smith completed a BA in European Studies from London Metropolitan University in 1995. He has taught English in Germany, Moscow and Saudi Arabia before returning to study at the University of Manchester. His PhD area is Contemporary US Foreign Policy, specifically the construction of a new grand strategic consensus in US foreign policy and national security strategy following September 11. He has been awarded an AHRC award and March–June 2006 was a Kluge Scholar at the Library of Congress, Washington, DC.

Emily Tanner is a Senior Researcher in the Quantitative Department of the National Centre for Social Research (NatCen). Her recent research projects include the National Adult Learning Survey, Study of Secondary School Admissions and the evaluation of the Adult Learning Grant. She has a DPhil from the University of Oxford (2005) where she investigated maternal employment, parenting and childcare in the Department of Social Policy and Nuffield College. Prior to doctoral study, Emily was a researcher at the Zigler Center for Child Development and Social Policy at Yale University.

Becky Tipper is a PhD student at the University of Manchester. Her research examines the relationships between children aged 7–11 and their pets – exploring the meanings that children give to these relationships, and the ways they take shape in children's everyday lives. From 2004 to 2006 she worked as a researcher on the ESRC-funded project 'Children Creating Kinship' at the University of Manchester. Becky previously studied Psychology (MA, University of St Andrews, 1999) and Social Research (MA, University of Leeds, 2003).

Justin Waring is a lecturer in medical sociology and health policy at the University of Nottingham. His primary research interests are in the changing character of medical professional work, culture and regulation. These interests have been developed within the context of the UK 'patient safety' agenda where he has considered how issues of error and risk are regulated, by both managers and medics, and interplay with notions of professionalism. After completing studies at the Universities of

Liverpool (1998) and Birmingham (1999), Justin undertook his PhD at the University of Nottingham between 2000 and 2003, followed by post-doctoral research at the University of Manchester.

Sheelah Flatman Watson is currently pursuing a PhD in Geography at NUI Maynooth. Her current research explores the spatial analysis of access to primary education for students with an intellectual and/or developmental disability, specifically the causal barriers to inclusion in mainstream and consequent outcomes of exclusion. Social justice, citizenship, equality, community and choice are the key elements that guide this work. Areas of interest and involvement include a local ARCH club, Special Olympics Network and local Autistic Children's Support Groups. Further areas of interest include behavioural psychology, learning styles, social and emotional skills development, relationships empathy and development of inclusive communities.

Kate Williams is a Research Fellow in the Centre for Criminal Justice Policy and Research at UCE Birmingham, following her PhD in criminology at Keele University. Kate's research interests include community involvement in policing, vigilantism and prostitution. Her work has recently appeared in the *Howard Journal of Criminal Justice* and commissioned research into resettlement has just been published by Government Office West Midlands. She is currently working on a joint-authored criminal justice textbook and an edited collection, amongst other projects. Kate also sits on the British Society of Criminology's Ethics and Professional Affairs Committee, together with the Executive Committee and Advisory Council.

Gina Wisker is Director of Learning and Teaching Development at Anglia Polytechnic University where she also coordinates women's studies and teaches English. Gina has supervised PhD and masters students for many years and now also researches postgraduate learning and supervisory practices and runs workshops on supervision and research methods. This has led to her writing *The Postgraduate Research Handbook* (Palgrave Macmillan, 2001) and *The Good Supervisor* (Palgrave Macmillan, 2005), along with a range of essays.

Introduction

About this book

This book aims to provide a resource to help research students through the process of accessing, undertaking and completing doctoral research in the social sciences and the humanities. The book seeks to realise this objective via a focus on research students' experiences, dilemmas, options and strategies in practice across a range of methodological, personal and institutional aspects of the doctoral process. While we felt that in the past few years there had been a welcomed burst of postgraduate and doctoral educational guides and detailed research methodology texts that debate the technical and analytical aspects of particular approaches, we identified a need for a textbook aimed at research students that does the following:

- Provides accessible advice and guidance across a spectrum of methodological, personal, emotional, practical and institutional issues suitable to an increasingly diverse student body.
- Provides an account of research as method, process and practice.
- Uses real life experiences to demonstrate the process of thesis development.

While research inquiries are informed by rigorous theoretical and methodological principles and plans, skill and craft progression is fundamentally developed via a process of applying these to real life circumstances and dilemmas. Research as it is practised remains under-reported for many reasons, and yet the novice seeking to develop into a professional researcher can potentially gain much from access to this level of practice and learning. For those embarking on independent academic research probably for the first time, there is huge scope for anxiety and uncertainty in seeking to apply the variety of theoretical, methodological and technical prescriptions to their specific research encounters. We sought to recognise the role of *learning by doing* within doctoral research by seeking to write a text that aimed to facilitate making informed choices and engagement with a range of research experiences and situations. We have included accounts from students to show how they managed the doctoral process, made strategic choices and developed their skills, as a means of contributing to the need to describe learning and research in practice.

The need for such a text was born from our concerns and considerations as recently graduated PhD students in addition to discussions about research dilemmas and support needs within broader peer and research methods networks. A brief overview of these motivating factors will help to set out for the reader our basic premises, the intended scope of the book and why the book is structured and written the way it is.

A gap in support for PhD students?

In their preface, Rugg and Petre (2004: vii) write:

> one of the most frequent laments of the postgraduate researcher is: 'Why didn't someone tell me that earlier?' They refer to what they call the *The Unwritten Rules of PhD Research* – rules, advice and guidance on a myriad of issues relating to the practice and culture of academia which aid the doctoral student in their progress. They also highlight that if key information is omitted from supervisory discussions or doctoral training this can potentially contribute to 'large amounts of confusion, depression, wasted effort and general tears and misery'. (Rugg and Petre, 2004: vii)

In their text, Rugg and Petre (2004) consider university doctoral procedures, the system of postgraduate education, networking, reading, writing, research design and publishing. They seek to impart their tacit knowledge of how to do the craft of academic research (such as developing your reading, writing and research design skills) as well as how to navigate and develop your academic career within university cultures and relationships. Such a sentiment also spurred us to write this textbook and, like Rugg and Petre, emerged from our own doctoral experience with critical concerns about the process.

We had other motivations too. We also wanted to acknowledge the growing diversity of the doctoral cohort and the need to recognise the connections between research as method, approach and principles. We wanted to focus on research as experienced and practised in specific ways by students engaged with real life situations, unexpected events and everyday institutional relationships. Our intention was to break down what can be alienating beliefs – that there is one right way to do research or one typical type of doctoral student and experience. There may well be 'hidden rules' that can help you progress but we felt recognition of students' capacities for applying their knowledge and awareness to the specific situations they faced was also needed in order to enhance motivations and resources for completion and researcher development.

The idea for this book emerged from our own experiences of grappling with undertaking doctoral research studies and applying our research training and knowledge to specific research problems. While we valued and utilised the range of theoretically and methodologically focused textbooks (with a particular interest in pursuing qualitative social science approaches), we felt that, first, there was a gap within the range of published research and method textbooks that provided generic accounts of putting research principles and plans into practice as a PhD student. We felt that beyond methodological debates that specifically addressed reflexivity within the research process or the application of specific approaches based on an examination of research as practice – there was little discussion of how research was actually conducted in real life situations. The problem with debates on reflexivity in research methods texts was that they were generally aimed at how to develop this particular methodology rather than speaking to researchers in general across disciplinary or methodological approaches. Yet we found that we valued, as did many of our peers, the sharing of our research dilemmas, issues and strategic thinking. We also felt that sharing how we were undertaking research in practice was a crucial aspect of relieving fears around 'doing things right' or overcoming isolation and worry within the doctoral process.

Secondly, we felt that the current range of textbooks and systems of support within universities (such as within supervisory teams and student support networks) often sustained a bounded notion of the researcher as devoid of other competing or personal commitments, concerns and demands. We concluded that despite the plethora of 'how to' manuals, there were few texts that really expressed the complexity of research experiences and the connections between your role as a researcher and your wider university and non-university life experiences. We felt that there needed to be more recognition that the PhD experience was more than theoretical and method-ological considerations – it was an experience that sat alongside another big experi-ence – *life*! Doing a PhD in the twenty-first century rarely follows the trajectory of undergraduate, masters and research degree without life interfering somewhere along the line. People do PhDs at all stages of life, with a whole manner of other commitments, burdens and work expectations that have to be managed. The PhD is increasingly difficult to fund, and if academia is the long-term career goal, then get-ting an academic post cannot be thought about when the viva is over. Further, the everyday nitty-gritty of doing doctoral research involves enhancing a rigorous social science approach while also contending with and managing multiple demands and responses both institutionally and personally.

We felt these two aspects of the PhD experience required more generic recog-nition. We hope to have brought together the process of learning to become an independent researcher through the application of method, principles and frame-works; and the embedded nature of research practice with other aspects of life expe-riences. We wanted to discuss an array of issues that research students negotiate, such as childcare, finance, emotional roller-coasters, personal challenges and personality clashes alongside a grounded discussion of the trials, tribulations and complexities of getting through designing, doing and writing a PhD. We hope overall to offer sup-port to doctoral students by providing descriptions of research in practice and a holistic view of the student experience – contributing to calls to demystify research and doctorates. Such a text can help the doctoral student exactly because as a novice researcher, confidence can be boosted through awareness that research in practice is a messy and diverse endeavour. Becoming a professional researcher involves engag-ing with this messiness and applying an approach that enhances research practice to maximise the possibilities presented. Doing a PhD is all about *learning through doing*, a process that can be enhanced by engaging with individual motivations, aspirations and specific research problems whilst utilising the available resources and opportunities at hand. It will probably mean making mistakes and being presented with unexpected outcomes and obstacles – requiring reflection and a perseverance to try something else or just try again! Learning, however, may be limited if research is thought of merely as the implementation of techniques leading students to fear if they are 'doing the right thing' or a 'good enough job'. These concerns need to be turned into a consideration of upholding research standards and rigour while expanding your skills and applications towards the numerous research dilemmas that can arise in practice.

To produce such a text we sought the input of a range of contributors – research students who themselves were in the throes of beginning or completing their doctorates. We wanted contributions from people at all stages of the PhD, a mix of those who had entered the process through traditional and non-traditional routes as well as at different stages of their own lifecourse. We wanted a good mix of disciplines from the social sciences and humanities that promoted a range of generic experiences across the subjects. The case study approach was decided as the most appropriate methodology because we wanted to show a range and variety of experiences, painting a realistic picture of the dilemmas and issues. We think we have done this because the contributions report on both mainstream and marginal perspectives. Some people who contributed were really struggling when they wrote their reflections; others had decided not to pursue the final stages of the PhD, whilst a few were starting new careers in academia and business after completing the process. Recruitment was through our own academic networks, advertisements on postgraduate networks and forums within our own university settings and beyond in the UK, inviting contributors to reflect on aspects of their experiences and research practices as students. We have also contributed to this process ourselves, drawing on our own PhD experiences.

Enhancing doctoral success: the changing shape of the PhD in the UK context

It is no coincidence that this book has emerged during a phase of reform and re-orientation within the UK doctoral system. The book, and its aims described above, indicates a growing concern with enhancing the doctoral experience, improving research practice and rates of completion. More people are undertaking doctoral research than ever before. The Higher Education Statistics Agency (2005) tells us that in 2004/05, 12,030 full time doctorate qualifications were awarded and a further 3,745 part time doctorates. These statistics represent a significant increase in people studying for doctorates in the UK. Ten years previous, in 1994/95 only 1,385 doctorates were awarded. This rise in student numbers has occurred alongside many changes and concerns surrounding doctoral education in the UK. Hockey's (1994) description of a PhD as a time of 'intellectual solitariness, individualistic and self autonomous' still holds true to some extent, but there have also been many changes that have altered the expectations, status and activities of PhD students. Doctoral students in the social sciences and humanities are increasingly contributing to undergraduate teaching, undertaking career development planning and are encouraged to develop a generic set of research skills. They are subject to new university procedures for on-going monitoring and target deadlines to meet completion projections (Harland and Plangger, 2004). Further, the idea of the 'typical' research student is becoming increasingly misleading, with many doctorates funded by external agencies, or as noted above, taken on a part-time basis.

Wider changes within and beyond Higher Education are driving developments in the PhD world. While there has been concern about standards of supervision and training within universities, there is also a debate about the role of undergraduate and postgraduate education in relation to the wider labour market and economic context. Universities have been under much pressure to re-organise and standardise doctoral education and supervision. At the same time the very purpose of a doctorate has become the subject of much debate.

Since the 1980s there has been concern at the length of time that students were taking to complete, as eight years was not uncommon, particularly in the social sciences and humanities. Sir Gareth Roberts was commissioned to carry out a review in the late 1990s in recognition of low submission rates (the Economic and Social Research Council (ESRC) submission rate was only 73% in 1994). These unacceptable levels of inefficiency were the target of radical changes, including:

- A four-year completion deadline.
- A managerial style of managing Higher Education.
- A need to establish a philosophy of apprenticeship for research rather than producing knowledge.
- Improvements and formalisation of training, supervision and guidance.
- Improvements of the 'throughput' of students, particularly from overseas.

The Roberts Review, entitled 'SET for Success' (2002), set out these plans and a vision for doctoral reform. Alongside the concern with non-completion and late submission, there were broader anxieties about the fit between the skills needed in the labour market and the quality of postgraduate students. There was concern that universities were not producing postgraduates with the necessary and adequate skills for a demanding twenty-first century international labour force. The PhD that was timeless, with no criteria for how long the exercise should take, was also a concern because it meant that students were out of the market place for longer and that their salaries were held down. This led to an overhaul in the training that postgraduates are given and a formalisation of the need for specific research methods training as part of the PhD package. The Roberts Review (2002) emphasised the need for universities to impart transferable skills to postgraduates who could then enter the labour market with a range of skills suitable for a variety of industries, not just academia.

Pre-empting the outcome of the Roberts Review, the four UK research funding councils produced a 'Joint Statement of UK Research Councils' (2001), which set out what is meant by training and transferable skills and includes the following categories:

- Research skills and techniques.
- Research environment.
- Research management.
- Personal effectiveness.
- Communication skills.
- Networking and team-working.
- Career management.

The ESRC introduced what is known as the 1+3 funding studentships which designated one year for formal training and an expectation that the PhD will be completed within the following three years. This is now recognised as the formal and common format for PhDs with a strong expectation that they are completed within the four-year period. Coupled with these changes, the Research Assessment Exercise and Quality Assurance Agency has also contributed to a regulated system of monitoring outputs, research activity and building research capacities.

These changes in the management and understanding of what a PhD is, have been met with criticisms that convey the continuation of diverse conceptions of the role and purpose of doctoral research. Leonard (2001: 23) suggests there are concerns with the approach of engineering doctoral studies in the following ways:

- Education at this higher level becomes no longer considered a welfare right or a path of self-development but part of the needs of industry and the employment market.
- The role of education to create a common culture or contribute to knowledge itself is undermined.
- The focus on training researchers through doctoral programmes reduces the aim of making a significant contribution to knowledge.

Despite these concerns though, the changes have contributed to new benchmarks for doctoral training and student development. Any student entering postgraduate study will realise they are being trained as a researcher as there is a heavy emphasis on learning research design, and qualitative and quantitative methods. There is improved supervision, both in terms of quality and accountability, as well as an emphasis on monitoring progress and tracking individuals through the system so they don't 'get lost'. An improvement in the Higher Education system as a whole is that of complaints procedures and Equal Opportunities mechanisms in an attempt to counterbalance the traditional prejudices that have long been associated with universities.

This text aims to recognise and further support agendas for widening participation, student development and doctoral completion via guidance covering a range of issues and experiences. The chapters set out below encourage students to think about their research problems, principles, objectives and resources and develop awareness suitable for a professional approach to research.

Personal development planning

We want to place this book in the wider context of Personal Development Planning (PDP hereafter), which is becoming an important aspect of Higher Education at both undergraduate and postgraduate levels. The Roberts Review 'Set for Success' urged funding councils to make sure that PhD programmes included a minimum of two weeks' dedicated training each year, based on developing research and transferable skills. To meet wider objectives of improving the standards of graduates with skills reaching beyond that of their expert subject, the PDP system was introduced in universities that took a keen interest in personal development.

In brief, the PDP is a process of structured activities and support whereby individuals reflect upon their learning, achievements and personal, education and career development (UK Grad Programme, 2004: 2–3). The process is often developed throughout the PhD but is kick-started in the first year. The types of activities include reviewing training needs; personal reflection and review; skills assessment; planning training; research log; collecting CV information and research planning. The benefits to those students who engage in the PDP process (currently it is largely voluntary) can include providing:

- A structured framework to reflect on personal and professional development.
- Empowerment for students to take control of their learning.
- Reflection on career management.
- Enhancement of the student progress monitoring process.
- Enhancement of project management, time management and goal setting skills.

The PDP process can effectively focus on employability, enabling students to:

- Record, reflect on and plan their own development.
- Highlight transferable skills.
- Make suitable career plans.
- Demonstrate employability.

Many of the chapters are written in the spirit of encouraging students to monitor their own development, plan for their success and troubleshoot where problems arise. We would encourage students to think about engaging with the PDP process in order to have structured time during the PhD to think constructively about their personal development alongside their intellectual abilities.

What this book does and does not do

This book seeks to:

- Provide strategies for thinking through common problems experienced by social science and humanities research students.

- Demystify the reality of doing a PhD via the use of real life student case studies of lived experiences.
- Balance a concern with rigorous research standards, student support and sustaining student well-being with a research–life balance.
- Contextualise research as involving practices, emotions, relationships and personal investments.
- Look beyond methodological and university agendas.
- Seek to address a broad range of issues for a broad student body.

The book aims to contribute to the wide-ranging literature on research methods and study strategies already available to research students. We believe there are many texts providing the following guidance and hence this book does not cover:

- In-depth guidance on particular methodological or design issues.
- Guidance on seeking doctoral funding.

Overview of chapters

The book is organised into four parts, the first two of which cover particular aspects of the research process while the second two focus more on the multiple roles of the doctoral student:

- Negotiating the research process.
- Writing, publishing and networking.
- Shifting identities and institutions.
- Relationships of support.

Part I discusses crucial aspects of beginning, designing and doing PhD research. The first chapter considers student motivations for doing doctoral research and illustrates not only the multiple routes into, and motivations for beginning a PhD, but also the role that our motivations play in the research process. Chapter 2 provides advice and case study accounts of moving from your initial research proposal towards a formulated, coherent and do-able research question. Chapters 3 and 4 consider experiences and options for establishing your supervisory team and engaging with ethical regulations for academic research. The final chapter in this part contemplates practices and strategies for data analysis.

Part II turns towards a focus on writing, networking and publishing. Chapter 6 specifically addresses aspects of writing as part of your thesis development and the process of writing up. Chapter 7 invites you to take your writing further, providing advice, case studies and encouragement in the publishing process. Chapter 8 takes a look at networking and the vital role that research relationships can play in the development of your ideas, career and skills.

The chapters written for Part III emphasise the connections between wider life experiences and research endeavours. Chapter 11 reviews some less traditional routes into PhD research and the challenges such routes can entail for both students and institutional change. One key aspect of change has been the increase in part–time doctorate programmes, which is further discussed in Chapter 12. Teaching has also become a central activity undertaken by doctoral students. Chapter 13 provides examples of how some students sought to extend their teaching skills and provides guidance on seeking adequate support and training alongside your research. Chapter 14 focuses on a major theme of the book, that of how research is intimately connected to emotional responses and orientations. Part IV reviews relationships of support. Chapter 15 examines the supervisory relationship and suggests a benchmark of what a student should receive in terms of supervision. Chapter 16 looks at the research and university environment in terms of its capacity to promote and inhibit the research process. Chapter 17 examines an increasing reality that many students who take a PhD are also parents and carers and must manage family commitments. Chapter 18 concludes the case studies by using the direct experiences of a university counsellor to highlight the role of counselling in the university context.

Part I
Negotiating the Research Process

The first part of the book introduces some of the questions that arise at the very early stages of thinking about doing a PhD and the steps necessary to find out about courses, institutions and supervisors. This section really is about 'negotiation' as this is at the heart of the induction phase into the PhD process and returning to education, which can be a daunting experience for many. In Chapter 1 we discuss some of the motivations that drive people to take on this task of producing an original piece of work in three years working full-time or six years part-time! Here we explore a range of motivations for doing the PhD and encourage you to choose a topic that will keep you fired up for the whole time. We hope this will clarify some of your own initial thoughts and also make you realise that the decision to do a PhD needs time as it is a significant life commitment. Chapter 2 deals with a question that has confused many students, including the authors, and is something that our own PhD students continually struggle with. It is not a simple process to pin your wide and general interests about a topic down to a research question that is focused and yet feasible. In this chapter we provide some broader understanding about the process of question formulation and offer some techniques for reducing down your ideas into a technical inquiry.

Chapter 3 is the first of two chapters that examines the relationship between the doctoral student and their supervisor (also see Chapter 15). Undoubtedly one of the most important aspects of conducting a PhD and yet sometimes the most anxious, we think about how you are allocated (or perhaps choose) an academic to supervise your work. Unpicking the many facets of the relationship, we acknowledge that changes in supervisors are sometimes inevitable and offer some solutions as to how to manage what can be an unsettling time. No doubt from undergraduate courses you will be aware that research is not conducted in a bubble, but that ethics is intrinsic to the research process. As postgraduates you need to take ethical issues within empirical research seriously, as your own research design will be scrutinised to assess whether it is ethical. In Chapter 4 contributors explain how ethics have affected their research, resulting in complex decisions, personal reflection and in some cases richer findings. At the heart of this chapter we explain more about the process of ethical governance which will affect students as they design and carry out research in the field.

The final chapter in Part I looks a little further into the doctoral process by asking 'What to do with your data?' Often students are so proficient at data collection and they amass so much information that they have problems making sense of it. This chapter provides techniques and suggestions for managing both qualitative and quantitative data, from preparing the data, familiarisation, coding and reading the findings. This is often a neglected stage in the data collection phase that is given little credence when students begin the doctorate. We hope we can get you to think about data analysis at an early stage as it is as important as formulating a question.

Chapter 1
Motivations for Doing a PhD

▶ The main motivations for doing a PhD
▶ Discussion of how topics are chosen
▶ A PhD as career development
▶ The personal agenda
▶ Tips on key questions to ask before applying

From our perusal of other 'how to' guides written for PhD students we have noted that not many pay attention to the initial motivations for doing a PhD. The reasons behind and pathways to considering and taking on board this endeavour are ultimately what will get you through the difficult patches. Here we explore some of the varied reasons why a PhD becomes a likely option and how subject topics are chosen. We asked the contributors to this book the following questions, which we urge you to ask yourself:

• What were your motivations for doing a PhD?
• How and why did you choose your topic?

We hope that you will take time to reflect on these questions and explore your own motivations for taking on a significant commitment that will put you in the privileged category of approximately 2% of the population who have achieved the highest qualification in the British education system.

So why bother?

Our contributors have provided us with the evidence to suggest there are five core reasons that motivate a PhD: career development; lack of job satisfaction; research as active engagement in politics; a personal agenda; and (sometimes) drifting into the challenge. These different motivating factors will be described through the narratives of the contributors.

Career development

One of the central motivating factors in taking on a PhD is to enhance career progression and development in existing and new occupations. Career development can be enhanced in several ways. For instance, you can already be in a job and consider this higher qualification as the route to quicker promotion, or specialisation. Or you could have reached a natural point in your career where progression to the next level would be smoother with a higher qualification. Sallyann Halliday describes how her desire to develop more critical skills through a concentrated period of research was identified as beneficial to her day job as a contract researcher:

> I felt that I had hit a 'turning point' in the work I was currently involved in as a contract researcher. For me, the motivation for doing a PhD was about being able to explore a topic I was really interested in through in-depth study, to widen my knowledge and develop different skills. I wanted to gain skills in critical thought and writing. Doing a PhD was the path I felt I should take and more importantly one I felt that I needed to go down to develop and progress further in my career (or possibly lead to a change in career focus). I saw it as a form of both personal and professional development.

For others, the desire to 'be an academic' meant that the PhD was an inevitable step into becoming a lecturer. Joseph Burridge speaks of how his desire to work in the university setting was the motivation for continually pursuing funding for a PhD:

> From the age of about fifteen I was sure that I wanted to pursue a career in academia, largely because of my love of reading and learning. A PhD was always going to be on the agenda, since it is no longer realistic to hope to begin such a career without one. I attempted to get funding immediately after finishing my first degree, but was unsuccessful and had to self-fund a masters degree as a means to demonstrate my seriousness for the next round of funding competitions. Fortunately it seemed to work and I was successful the second time around!

Self-funding a one-year postgraduate course is a popular method of finding out whether further study is the right route. Although this is a financial cost, part-time study is always an option before making a big life change by fully committing to a PhD. However, it is not always the case that a PhD 'was on the cards' in a person's life pathway. Sometimes wider dissatisfaction or a desire for another challenge can prompt enrolment onto a PhD programme.

Lack of job satisfaction

While taking on board a PhD can be born out of developing a career path, at the same time a lack of job satisfaction in current employment can be a motivating factor to seek an alternative enterprise. Melanie Shearn describes how dissatisfaction in her employment, coupled with some wider life goals, naturally led her to consider a PhD:

> I had worked in a number of different jobs in related industries and found that I lacked job satisfaction. I wanted to do something that made, in my view, a contribution to society. But so did other people and competition for these jobs was fierce. It seemed to me that the only way to make up for a lack of particular life experiences was to have substantive knowledge and expertise of a topic area. I also really enjoyed querying things and providing answers or direction. I thought that a PhD could combine my substantive interests with research skills.

BOX 1.1 Don't enter into a PhD lightly

Make sure you understand the commitment, and try to determine whether you need the PhD to fulfil your career objectives. Also, be honest with yourself – are you *really* interested in the subject? Do you *really* have a burning curiosity to find out the answers to your questions? [Martin Smith]

Personal agenda

Often it is personal motivations that inspire people to investigate a specific topic or gives them the desire to take on the job of giving voice to marginalised groups, or in some way they want to set the record straight against tides of stereotypes and misinformation that can spuriously inform our understanding of the world. Personal insights or close contact with certain groups, lifestyles or experiences are familiar reasons for pursuing further studies in the social sciences and humanities. Below, Sonali Shah reflects on how her own experiences as an Asian woman living with a physical impairment led her to study for a PhD:

I applied for a journalism course, passed the entrance exam and was also given a bursary. However, I was not given a place because the employers thought that my disability would prevent me from achieving and coping with the work required. This was seen as a significant turning point in my future professional orientation. It was this and previous experiences of disability discrimination, coupled with the Asian achievement-oriented culture within which I was brought up, that influenced my decision to pursue academic research to investigate what makes a disabled high-flyer.

No doubt you will meet people with interesting personal connections to their PhD topic and fieldwork site. This can often be an inspirational motivation to take the PhD forward and manage those difficult barriers to getting the job done.

Research as politics

Closely tied to personal experiences, political principles and everyday politics that influence policy and shape our lives, as well as world events, can also be triggers for pursuing further studies. Joseph Burridge describes how his wider interest in political controversies shaped his motivations and ideas for a PhD:

I had always been interested in controversy and argumentation since it seems to me that they are fairly fundamental to the way in which we relate to one another as human beings socially and politically. I had planned to undertake a more extensive and detailed analysis of the political debate over the repeal of Section 28 – a piece of legislation which has now been repealed but is usually described as having banned the 'promotion of homosexuality' – which had been the topic of my masters thesis. However, as I was finishing the thesis, the events of 11th September 2001 took place, and the aftermath seemed to be a location in which I could pursue some similar themes to those that had interested me about Section 28.

PhDs are not isolated events that exist between the individual, the supervisor and the research subjects. Real life events, political change and the localised and globalised setting of the topic have bearing on motivations as well as the trajectory of the content of the research.

Drifting In

The final factor is not as consciously driven as some of the above reasons for pursuing PhD study. Several contributors described how they drifted into a PhD after undergraduate or postgraduate studies. This notion of drift is not necessarily something we would discourage, as, after all, none of us knows what opportunities are around the corner and we cannot all have clearly thought-out plans from the start. Yet we would add a cautionary tale to those scenarios that lead to individuals drifting into a PhD without giving very careful consideration to the entity that is being taken on. Martin Smith spent several years working towards his doctorate but in the end discontinued his studies as the need to earn cash took over. Martin remarks below on the dangers of drift:

> I somewhat drifted into doing a PhD, in a subject area that was of interest to me, but was not my academic passion. I was unprepared for the challenge and commitment I needed to make in the years to come, and feel now that I should have taken a masters course to see whether higher level research and study was for me.

The reality is that personal circumstances are a clear indicator as to whether a PhD is viable in terms of a drop in earnings, the prospects of the market place after completion and the opportunities that are available. Bill Armer, an older student who returned to education late, describes how his options after his undergraduate degree were fairly limited, and hence the 'drift' into further study:

> As a late returner to education, I had no clear motivation when I first undertook my BA degree. Finding myself unemployed and potentially unemployable, I really drifted into academia as an honourable alternative to the dole.

Ultimately the motivations for undertaking a PhD span the spectrum of the personal and the political, motivated by the subject or a specific project, influenced by a role model or attracted by the department, institution or even the student lifestyle! Often, career plans are somewhere in the complexities of motivations as students wrestle with the question 'Where will having a PhD get me?'

Choosing the topic (or does the topic choose you?)

An intriguing aspect of doing a PhD is the plethora of topics that people choose. One of the attractive aspects of doctoral studies is the freedom of topic and area of study, as long as the end product fulfils the criteria of originality and a contribution to knowledge. Critics suggest a change is taking place in the types of PhDs that are funded as topics are influenced by the interests of research councils, who determine which areas should receive priority funding. How people select their research topics could take the length of this book alone, as there are a myriad of reasons that involve the personal and the political as well as the rather ordinary and mundane.

Strategies of deduction

The desire to do a PhD can sometimes precede the topic of interest. It is not always the case that the topic of interest is the driving force behind wanting to study for at least three years. There can be other strategies of deduction that provide a clear direction in terms of discipline and topic. Melanie Shearn decided that a PhD was what she wanted to do before the topic was obvious:

> I drew up lists of all the things I was passionate about in the world, as well as some of the things I wanted to do in my life. I merged these and came up with a topic on which I based a research funding proposal.

Similarly, it can be the case that you are clear about the general area in which you want to study, but are not quite sure about the actual topic or how to develop a succinct research idea and set of questions. Often this entanglement can be ironed out with some 'thinking' sessions with your supervisor. Before starting the PhD, Sharon Elley had worked as a youth worker and was particularly interested in exploring young people's experiences of relationships but was not quite sure which angle to take. Finding a gap in the literature was a key factor. Finally, having some contact with professionals that designed and implemented the sex education programme, it was decided that this is where the gap in knowledge lay and a feasible study was designed.

Job interest

Just as a desire for career progression or career change can motivate a PhD, developments, knowledge and areas of interest you are exposed to in the work setting can be the inspirational factor for your choice of topic. Richard Heslop had been a policeman for twenty years before deciding to turn a work-based topic into a research question:

> My original plan was to apply to research for a PhD in the field of politics and policing. However, around that time my career took a change of direction and I was posted into the Force Training Department. Working as a trainer was perhaps the most rewarding role I had ever had in the police service and it sparked a strong academic interest in adult education.

The change in Richard's day job (police work) was significant as it meant that instead of a traditional PhD, a professional doctorate in education (Ed.D) was more appropriate. Relationships with employers and the work-base settings are increasingly important if studying for a PhD part-time whilst still working. You may be directly relating your PhD questions to the work setting, using contacts at work as gatekeepers or work-based resources to access key informants and respondents.

Politics and passion

Invariably you will find that people who are studying or have achieved a PhD are passionate about their topic. If they are not when they start out, they often become emphatic defenders of their territory by the end, after living, sleeping and breathing the stuff for three years (or more!). Passion for a topic and the politics that often surround the topic, are strong motivating forces for embarking on knowledge production. Teela Sanders chose to study the female sex industry after directly working with sex workers as a welfare professional and experiencing disillusionment with an academic literature that did not appear to reflect the reality of some aspects of the sex industry. JK Tina Basi demonstrates below how her own personal history was related to her desire to pursue a certain line of inquiry about a specific group of people:

> My motivation to do the PhD was born out of a desire to produce more knowledge about Indian women. I was tired of always being told how Indian girls should be and the things that they should not be doing. I wanted to find out for myself what women in India were up to. However, I knew that to make it credible I couldn't just 'hang out' in India; I had to tie my curiosity in with an ongoing dialogue. Thus a feminist research project on Indian women's identities was born.

Our passion for the topics we choose is not always clear cut from the start but is vaguely in the background of a number of activities we undertake. It can be at the point of thinking about a significant piece of work such as a PhD that these ideas can become solidified. Bill Armer, who had skirted around the topic of disability and eugenics for several years, describes this natural process of arriving at a topic:

> At the heart of my PhD research topic was the interplay between eugenics and genetics, which was sheer self-indulgence. Since childhood in the 1950s, when the topic was fresh in the societal memory, I have been both repelled and fascinated by the horrors of Nazi Germany. I have, it seems forever, been vaguely aware of the dangers of eugenics. I never intended to develop an academic interest here, but looking back it was almost inevitable that I would.

There are often underlining reasons, whether personal, political or a combination of both, that usually motivate people to want to know more. While this is not something that can be measured in an interview, or can be assessed through a research proposal, the desire to want to study this very narrow and specialised area for at least three years has to be something you are very clear about. Martin Smith ended up with a research topic that he was only mildly interested in, and he recounts below how this was not enough to keep him motivated when faced with dilemmas:

> My choice of topic was not founded on having a deep interest in any particular topic, which in hindsight I see as a mistake. At the end of the day, the drive to complete the PhD has to come from oneself. It's hard to work in the library until late at night on a topic you don't really enjoy when there's always the alternative of the College bar.

Potentially the trickiest part of the PhD is taking the plunge and saying 'yes' this is something I want to do and feel passionate enough about to make significant sacrifices. PhDs do mean making changes in your personal, social and work life and therefore those initial decisions should be carefully considered.

BOX 1.2   Are you passionate about your subject?

Ask yourself:

- Does your interest in the area relate closely to your personal experiences, political viewpoint or professional concerns?
- Do you hold opinions or motives that shape how you are looking at the issue in a particular way?
- What are the implications for your research questions?
- Do your interests and experiences lead you to ask specific questions?
- What alternative questions can be asked?

Key Points to Remember

▶ There are no correct reasons for doing a PhD but think carefully about 'why'.
▶ If career development is the main motivation, assess what the PhD will give you.
▶ Personal or political motivations are common but these must be balanced by genuine academic interest.
▶ Passion for your subject is an important ingredient for success and stamina – make sure you have this at the start.

SUGGESTED READING AND RESOURCES

Bentley, P.J. (2006) *The PhD Application Handbook*. Maidenhead: Open
  University Press.
Etherington, K. (2004) *Becoming a Reflexive Researcher: Using Ourselves in
  Research*. London: Jessica Kingsley.
Gordon, A.V. (2005) *MBA Admissions Strategy: From Profile Building to
  Essay Writing*. Maidenhead: Open University Press.
Walliman, N.S.R. (2005) *Your Research Project: A Step-by-Step Guide for the
  First Time Researcher.* London: Sage.
Wilkinson, D. (2005) *The Essential Guide to Postgraduate Study*. London:
  Sage.

National Postgraduate Committee—www.npc.org.uk
UK Grad programme—www.grad.ac.uk

Chapter 2
Formulating a Research Question

Moving from the initial research proposal towards a formulated research question

Chapter 1 considered a variety of routes into, and motivations for, doctoral research. Another difference at the outset of your research can be the degree of autonomy you have in devising your focal research questions and the degree of prior research undertaken in your doctoral research area. You may have become familiar with, and deeply interested in, your research area over many years of undergraduate and postgraduate education, gaining funding from a research council. Alternatively, you may be undertaking a PhD as part of a wider research project. Here, you may have less autonomy in devising your focal research questions and be accountable to an external funder as well as your university. You may also be undertaking doctoral research that involves venturing into new research areas compared with your previous academic interests. However, across this spectrum of circumstances, the beginning of your doctoral research is likely to involve a period of immersion and focusing as you move from a research title and general proposal to a set of formulated, coherent and do-able research questions. Even within studies that have been commissioned by outside agencies or designed prior to your involvement, it is likely you will need to spend time understanding the wider context of your team project and refining your focal PhD research questions. This period has been described as a period of 'reducing uncertainty' (Phillips and Pugh, 2005), 'progressive focusing' (Arksey and Knight, 1999) and 'generating an appropriate and coherent research problem' (Punch, 2000). This initial stage combines excitement when beginning your project, uncertainty in getting to know a new area or taking your knowledge to a more critical level as well as learning the skills and process of 'research problem formulation'. Focusing towards a coherent and do-able research problem that contributes to the building of knowledge in your area is a challenging task. John Roberts was interested in the general topic of 'free speech in public spaces' but found the task of focusing his research 'one of the most daunting tasks he faced' during his PhD research. We hope you can retain your enthusiasm and interest in your research topic while persevering and selectively focusing down your study appropriately for doctoral research.

The need to focus your research and generate a coherent research problem cannot be stressed enough. Central research questions, hypothesis or problems give your research activities purpose and direction, linking your research to an ongoing debate and/or body of knowledge. Without an explicitly formulated and worked through purpose or focus (or at least a preliminary one) your research project is likely to get steered in all sorts of directions. Without a formulated and feasible set of questions you risk:

- Feeling overwhelmed by your research.
- Feeling uncertain about the value of your research.
- Feeling unclear about what you are doing and where you are heading.
- Duplicating previous research.
- Asking common sense questions.
- Feeling uncertain about the wider academic significance or placing of your research.
- Generating data that is too general or vague and therefore difficult to draw conclusions from.

Research questions do not often appear in a sudden brain-wave! Rather, they are generated through a process of engaging with your research topic or interests (which may of course lead to some brain-wave ideas). This engagement can involve analysing and thinking about previous work in your area or undertaking a period of initial data collection. The former approach involves deductively generating research questions as you are deducing some focal questions from thinking about existing empirical and theoretical developments in your research area and identifying the gaps, ambiguities and inconsistencies within previous work. The latter approach involves inductively generating research questions from a period of data collection – looking afresh at a research topic or social phenomena. Many studies in practice involve a mixture of deductive and inductive approaches (see Blaikie, 2000). Research questions are therefore 'formulated' through an ongoing process of engagement with your research interests, setting and/or prior research.

Distinguishing between research title, research area, general and focal research questions

What is a 'formulated' research question? Drawing on her own research and supervisory background, Gina Wisker advises students to distinguish between the research title, focal area and key research questions (also see Phillips and Pugh, 2005; Punch, 2000). Problems arise if students persist in thinking that their doctoral research title and general research area also convey their research questions, as the latter are much more focused and specific. Gina illustrates the role of these different aspects of your research proposal:

(1) *Project title*:   This is a precise statement about the research aims and area. An example would be: 'A study of the effects of research development programmes on postgraduate student learning'. You will then need to generate research questions indicating the specific ways you will contribute to this area.

(2) *A field of study*:   This is much broader than a project title such as 'postgraduate student learning'. In defining your research area you will need to think about what is your broad area and what are the boundaries of your research area and what is excluded.

(3) *Overall research questions*:   This defines what you are asking and finding out about. For example: 'How and in what ways do the current UK and Australian research development programmes focus on and contribute to the development of postgraduate student learning and research higher degree success?'

(4) *Focal research questions*:   Your overall research question then needs to be broken down into focal research questions which provide a clear link to your data generation or empirical and theoretical analysis.

The chapter now turns to some strategies that may help you to comprehensively formulate your research area, title and questions.

Gaining an overview of the literature and research

Gaining an overview of the theoretical and empirical debates in your research area will generate an understanding of previous research and dominant approaches. Whether you are inductively or deductively generating your focal research questions, getting to know previous research in your area will help you to identify gaps in prevailing knowledge. In the early stages of her doctoral research, Harriet Churchill spent much time 'immersing herself in the literature'. Her supervisors had advised her to read around her research area and identify some 'gaps in knowledge'. In hindsight, Harriet felt it took her a year or so to demystify this process. Later on in the research process, Harriet developed strategies that aid thinking about previous knowledge via gaining an overview of a research area. These consisted of identifying seminal works and literature overviews, thinking about the research approaches and questions that have been developed, devising ways of presenting research and popular debates using diagrams or charts and asking her supervisors about key empirical and theoretical contributions.

BOX 2.1   Gaining an overview of the literature relevant to your research area

Ask yourself:
- What previous research has been conducted?
- What have been the main research questions?
- What kinds of questions have been asked, i.e. descriptive, explanatory or exploratory?
- What has the previous research concluded?
- What have been the main approaches/perspectives within previous research?
- What are the key concepts and conceptual debates?
- What debates/writers/topics or approaches interest me most?
- Are there any empirical gaps in the area?
- Are there any underdeveloped or less utilised approaches?

Strategies for gaining an overview may include:
- Regularly review your detailed reading notes with a view to seeking to identify common research questions, approaches and claims across studies.
- Use speed and scan reading to gain an overview of a text.
- Identify literature reviews and area overviews.
- Identify seminal work.
- Map out key methodological approaches to date.
- Seek to identify and define key concepts in your research area.
- Map out theoretical differences between studies.
- Use tables/charts/diagrams to summarise large amounts of information.

Sonali Shah was faced with the need to re-design her doctoral study once she discovered her initial proposal was not original or appropriate, a process that involved much uncertainty and anxiety:

The direction of my research changed somewhat after a literature search. I realised that my original research topic had been investigated before, I would not be adding anything new to knowledge. This led to fear about what my research would be. It was a combination of my supervisor lending me a book and thinking about the gaps in the research done in my area that prompted my final PhD direction. I reformulated my research questions around a study on investigating what influences career development and success for disabled people. I was very enthusiastic about this, especially since much of the existing research in relation to the employment of disabled people tended to focus either on their under-employment or unemployment. I was encouraged that I would definitely be contributing something new to knowledge.

Sonali demonstrates a systematic approach to devising her research questions. The process of engaging with the previous research in her area led her to abandon her initial research area. However, with persistence, critical thinking and support from her supervisor, she was able then to identify a fruitful gap in existing knowledge which provided the basis for an alternative research design.

Generating research questions from a period of data collection

An inductive approach to formulating your general and focal research questions can involve focusing one's questions after an initial period of fieldwork (Mason, 2002). Some qualitative ethnographic approaches, for example, aim to generate questions following a period of 'immersion' in the research setting. The aim is to link your questions more to the prominent issues and themes arising from the research setting or lived experience rather than from prior academic research knowledge, popular social representations or even the researcher's own preconceptions (see Atkinson et al., 2001; Crang and Cook, 2006; Mason, 2002 for ethnographic approaches). However, make sure you have a clear rationale and timeframe for preliminary fieldwork. Several of our contributors noted the complexity of managing this phase and approach. They discussed the need to be quite strict on the time allowed for this initial period of 'exploration' and quite disciplined in ensuring they did go on to focus their research in specific ways. Part of the problem could be that you need to think further about what is required and feasible for doctoral research. The next four sections consider prominent issues in research question formulation: quantitative research questions; questions that are too vague; questions that are too restrictive; feasibility issues and 'originality'.

Common issues in research question formulation

Thinking quantitatively

Whether your intended research project will use qualitative or quantitative research methods, or a mixed approach, the process of finalising a set of research questions is similar. Quantitative approaches, however, are suited to asking particular questions leading to the generation of quantitative data and the analysis of such data. Blaikie (2003: 11) describes the process as follows:

- **The research problem**: This is generally a very broad problem, such as 'the apparent lack of concern about environmental issues among many people and the unwillingness of many to act responsibly with regard to these issues'. This is too broad and unwieldy as it stands, so must be reduced down to some coherent and measurable questions.
- **The research questions**: These are needed to turn the broad research problem into a researchable set of questions. For instance: (1) To what extent is environmentally responsible behaviour practised? (2) Why are there variations in the levels of environmentally responsible behaviour?
- **The research objectives:** Each question must then be reduced to another set of objectives in order to explore, describe, understand, evaluate or assess the social phenomena.
- **What data can be collected:** Deciding what empirical evidence can be collected has a significant bearing on the final formulation of questions and objectives. You need to ask: What can realistically be observed? How can data be recorded? How can the data be analysed?

Is your question too vague?

Having a research question that is excessively broad or too vague is a common problem among doctoral students. Often this situation merely means that further 'progressive focusing' needs to occur. There needs to be further thinking through of vague questions to turn them into more focused ones. Gina Wisker, Harriet Churchill and John Roberts all felt that, on reflection, their PhD research questions remained too vague for too long. Working with vague questions led them to amass a huge amount of data, some of which they did not have time to analyse. It took Gina eighteen months to arrive at a 'formulated research question'. Harriet and John undertook some fieldwork before they focused their research questions. Harriet felt that, in hindsight, her research could have been more focused in the initial stages. In practice, Harriet focused her research quite a lot during the data analysis and writing up stages:

The research, looking at lone mothers' experiences of caring and providing for children at a time of national policy change in supporting parenting and parental employment, could have been enhanced by a more focused approach earlier on. There were many facets to the final thesis – some of which I could have focused on more – such as professional discourses on parents' support needs, mothers' concerns around parenting, mothers' strategies for financially providing for their children and so on. Having quite broad research questions meant that a lot of 'focusing the research' actually occurred in data analysis and writing phases – however by then I was already restricted by the data I had and lacked the time to focus in some of the directions I wanted to (because this would have required more data collection). Overall, though, by the end of my thesis I had a much more comprehensive picture of the research area, and now I feel more able to generate focused research questions.

John Roberts also took the approach of 'letting a focus emerge' from his field-work. However, a problem for John was that he gathered a lot of data covering a broad theoretical focus, which he did not have the time to analyse within his doctoral research. Some of his data did alternatively provide useful material, though, for subsequent publications and research:

My original research title was to conduct an ethnographic study of Speaker's Corner. I aimed to immerse myself in its everyday activities in order to understand the various social processes and relationships (i.e. how the audience, speakers and policy behave) that contribute towards, and help reproduce, its identity as a place for free speech. So I entered the research field with a vague idea. However, this had not yet been formulated into one definable research question. Two further turning points occurred. First, I stumbled over a brilliant social history book that described an earlier version of Hyde Park Corner speeches. I then set out to trace the history of public speaking at Hyde Park. Second, I discovered a whole wealth of historical information about the regulation of public speaking in the nineteenth and twentieth centuries at Hyde Park at Kew Public Records Office. Later on though only one area of data informed my thesis, the other areas informed subsequent journal articles.

Is your research question too narrowly defined or restrictive?

At the other end of the spectrum is the problem of your questions being too restrictive. This is a problem whereby questions are too loaded with prior assumptions and common sense connections that explanatory capacity becomes restricted. As a supervisor, Gina Wisker often encourages students to 'unpack questions that are too narrowly defined' for the purpose of a PhD. Gina gives the example of a student seeking to establish 'How and why do girls fail in school?' This question begins with 'too many assumptions that have not been critically subjected to rigorous analysis':

> This research question already gives the sense of a fore-grounded conclusion – that girls fail in school – thus the question from the outset rejects a body of contradictory evidence and closes off explanatory avenues. In this case the student needs to read more about this topic carefully to identify the debates in the area and a gap in knowledge rather than going over old ground. He needs to ask more open questions of the research area and population rather than prejudging and so narrowing responses and interactions into a pre-determined focus.

In this case, Gina facilitated a critical analysis of the literature and research in the area by helping her student to devise 'a kind of matrix to describe and evaluate the ways in which previous authors were exploring and engaging with the issues'. Then 'from this analysis of previous research we generated an appropriate research question' – one that 'goes beyond an initial exploratory statement' and one that gets to the 'heart of the work, the issues, the concerns – so that theories interrogate and scaffold the exploration and questioning'.

BOX 2.2   Unpacking your research question

Ask yourself:

- Do my questions pre-suppose any explanatory relationships?
- Do my questions uphold any assumptions about the research area? On what basis are these sound? Is there any contradictory evidence?
- Do my questions make assumptions about cause and effect relationships? Are these relationships disputed by any research?
- Do my research questions indicate a particular theoretical or methodological approach? What other theories and approaches in the area are there?
- What do others such as my supervisor think about my questions?

Is your question going to facilitate an original contribution to knowledge?

Harriet Churchill felt her PhD research suffered from a lack of focal research questions. Later on in her study she felt if she had focused her research more after some preliminary analysis of early interviews she could have generated a more 'original' research project. In the final data analysis stage, Harriet realised her initial interviews raised what could have been some more original lines of inquiry. However, Harriet reflects that changing her research question and following new leads in the early stages of her PhD felt like having to 'start again' or take a step backwards.

Making an original contribution to knowledge certainly can be a tough criterion to meet within doctoral research. However, originality is likely to emerge through the ongoing process of deeply engaging with an area of interest and your research activities. Gina Wisker describes how her PhD students often experience a 'learning leap' that occurs in the latter stages of generating a thesis. This 'learning leap' is where the 'real question or real contribution to knowledge emerges in the later stages of the thesis'. After this 'leap' there is a kind of conceptual penny-drop phase that brings the thesis together and 'work starts to be theorised and conceptualised in more complex and coherent ways'. The student begins to develop their capacities for making a contribution to understanding and knowledge in their subject area.

What is important is to try not to dwell on nor deny these 'problems or concerns' but to seek to establish whether your aims are too broad or vague or narrow and to seek ways to appropriately focus and justify your research. If you feel unsure of your focus, find it difficult to articulate or establish where your study fits into a wider picture of academic knowledge – then you will need to continue with the process of turning your 'general enthusiasm' for a subject into a 'clearly defined research project' guided by clearly formulated questions. The emphasis here is on the continual and active engagement on the part of the researcher with the issues of originality and prior knowledge – indicating that questions neither fall from the sky nor suddenly hit us in a moment of *Eureka!* clarity. Rather, they are formulated through a process of thinking about your research area, interests and design.

Thinking about feasibility

Phillips and Pugh (2005) found that PhD students often under-estimate how much time and effort is required for each stage of the research process and for their overall project. Thinking about, and getting advice on, the 'do-ability' of your research project will be an important aspect of devising your research questions and approach.

BOX 2.3   Thinking about feasibility

This is about linking the **aims of your project** with the **requirements of a PhD** and the **resources available** to you for your doctoral studies.

Ask yourself:

- What is required from doctoral research? (e.g. ask your supervisor, read your university regulations)

- What resources are available to support my research? (e.g. time, IT, training support, conference budget)
- Do I have any particular constraints to consider? (e.g. other commitments, lack of resources, part-time enrolment, juggling a research job with PhD research)

The fit between your research questions and overall design

As you generate your general and focal research questions, you will also be thinking about your research design as a whole. In moving to your overall research design you will then need to specify the theoretical and methodological frameworks to your study. The main principles guiding your design are to ensure a consistent fit between your research questions, your methodological and theoretical approach and the resources and requirements for undertaking your PhD research. This consistency directly relates to producing a valid and effective research design. You need to ensure that you are able to fulfil the requirements for doctoral research and able to complete the study within the deadline required (Mason, 2002). The following two boxes identify some of the crucial considerations in research design. These issues are covered widely in the research methods literature and some useful resources are given below.

BOX 2.4 Ontological and epistemological underpinnings to your research

In thinking about your general research area and what you wish to find out about – you will need to think about your underlying ontological and epistemological frameworks. Your **ontology** relates to what you are identifying as social reality and what we think social reality consists of. For example, are you wanting to examine decisions, identities, institutions, discourses or experiences? All of these concepts refer to different 'things' and you need to think about what you think these concepts represent. Think about:

- What is the nature of social phenomena indicated by our research area, title and questions?
- What alternative representations of reality could we envisage?
- How am I conceptualising social phenomena?
- How are these conceptualisations contested in the social sciences?
- How do these conceptualisations inform my methodological approach?

(Continued)

(Continued)

Your **epistemological** stance relates to how you conceptualise knowledge and your underlying theory of knowledge:

- What do you consider to be evidence of the social realities defined above?
- How do you envisage gaining 'knowledge' about them?

You are likely to return to these questions many times during your research! (see Blaikie, 2000; Mason, 2002).

Key Points to Remember

▶ Formulating a research question emerges from the process of engaging with the debates, knowledge and approaches in your research field.
▶ Seek ways of gaining an overview of your area.
▶ Ask yourself what have been the dominant theoretical, empirical and methodological approaches in your research area.
▶ Seek feedback on your research questions – ask yourself and others if your questions are too broad or restrictive.
▶ Think about the links between your research question (as content and type) and the possible theoretical and methodological approaches you can take.

SUGGESTED READING

Blaikie, N. (2000) *Designing Social Research: The Logic of Anticipation.* Malden: Polity Press.

Creswell, J.W. (2002) *Research Design: Qualitative, Quantitative and Mixed Method Approaches.* London: Sage.

Mason, J. (2002) *Qualitative Researching*, 2nd edn. London: Sage.

Punch, K.F. (2000) *Developing Effective Research Proposals.* London: Sage.

Saunders, M., Lewis, P. and Thornhill, A. (2003) *Research Methods for Business Students,* 3rd edn. Upper. Saddle River, NJ: Prentice-Hall.

Chapter 3
Choosing and Changing Supervisor

What this Chapter Includes:

▶ Insights into the nature of the supervisor–student relationship
▶ Suggestions on how to make the right choice first time
▶ Details of common problems that occur in the relationship
▶ Reasons for seeking to change your supervisor
▶ Suggestions how to do this both informally and formally
▶ The process of finding a new supervisor

Making the right choice

Your relationship with your supervisor is probably the most crucial variable that will affect how you experience the PhD journey, your intellectual development and indeed whether you submit on time. All of the study guides include chapters offering copious insights and direct advice about managing your supervisor. We suggest you familiarise yourself with these too, as the more preparation for this interesting relationship the better. However, often little importance is attached to specifically discussing how you end up with a supervisor, and also what to do when things go wrong. This chapter therefore deals with the early stage of finding or being allocated a supervisor and pre-empting any difficulties that may arise.

The level of control you have over choosing your supervisor may vary. There are normally two processes whereby you obtain a supervisor. The more traditional route is that on application to a department you are allocated a supervisor based on a suitable match of academic expertise with your proposed area of work. Many institutions operate a system of joint supervision – one person is appointed as the 'lead' and another the 'second' supervisor. Often this is an advantage because you can demand two people's time and attention instead of one! It also means that when one takes time out for whatever reason you still have another supervisor to consult. There are also downsides to this system though, as three people in the relationship can be crowded, especially if the two academics have polarised views on how your PhD should be conducted. In these scenarios it is often a case of allowing them to squabble amongst themselves!

The second process of obtaining a supervisor is one that relies on you proactively seeking out individuals that you want to work with. This approach is described by Claire Maxwell:

> I developed a research proposal based on my MSc thesis. From the research proposal I was able to identify the 'experts' in the field who were based at universities in the region where I lived. I sent my proposal and CV via email to the three or four academics and one potential supervisor got back to me almost immediately, offering to meet to discuss my proposal further.

Whether you are aware of whom you would like to work with or whether you are happy to let the institution take care of the allocation, this chapter will equip you with a basic framework to assess whether the supervisor is the right match for you.

The ingredients of a successful relationship

Clearly the first ingredient of a wholesome and productive relationship with a mentor relates to the extent to which their academic expertise matches your own initial interests. Because PhD topics are so specific, do not expect an identical match (a supervisor who is too close to your exact topic can also be far too competitive) but instead look for someone who is generally in your subject area. Looking for a generic specialist will also increase your scope of institutions, particularly if your family circumstances commit you to a certain locality. Once likely mentors have been identified, simply make direct contact by emailing your CV and a research proposal (make this concise – two A4 pages for example). This will start off the process of application and a phase of both parties checking out suitability.

When you are called for an interview or indeed offered a place, other points to consider are the department's rating in the Research Assessment Exercise (which measures research excellence against a criterion), the facilities for postgraduates (such as a computer, office space, conference grants, library account, photocopying allowance) and the general atmosphere of the environment.

- How will you be able to support me if your area of expertise is not that related to my PhD research?
- How many students have you supervised?
- How do they see the role of the supervisor?
- What could I expect? [Claire Maxwell]

When selecting or being allocated a supervisor, of great concern to students is the extent to which the academic has supervised before. Of course, an academic with a track record of students submitting in good time, passing their viva and going on to have a healthy career is an advantage, but do not dismiss younger, less experienced academics. Their closeness to the PhD experience is added value, plus they will be more clued up on the changing nature of the PhD, which can be used to your advantage. Also, more junior staff will probably have more time than senior academics who are over-burdened with commitments, many of which take them away from the university. It is worth pointing out also that academics who take on PhD candidates are bound by systems that check their performance, making sure that their quality of supervision reaches the appropriate standard and that they are steering the student in the right direction.

Three contributors have described the third ingredient, personal compatibility, as the most important aspect of the supervisor–student relationship. It can be the make-or-break element of the PhD experience. Although it is difficult to assess how much you will 'gel' with a person on the basis of a few meetings, this element requires making an early judgement call.

BOX 3.2

Bill Armer, a mature PhD student who did not have a successful first supervisory relationship, summarises the mission to find a suitable supervisor: 'What you are looking for is a person with whom you can "do business" on a personal level.'

You may be allocated a supervisor who works in an area that is not directly the same as yours. Sometimes this is not problematic but there are times when this lack of specialisation can be a cause for concern. Sonali Shah expressed concerns regarding her allocated supervisor:

> I have always been confused with regards to the basis on which my supervisor was selected as there seemed to be a mismatch of methodological interests. Her background was in quantitative research and I wanted to develop skills in qualitative research. The second concern was that my supervisor's field of expertise was nothing to do with disability, which was a primary factor in my research. Moreover she was more of a 'teaching academic' rather than a 'research academic'.

Sonali's case covers a wide range of concerns relating to who mentors you through the process and demonstrates what scenarios could have been grounds for seeking an alternative supervisor. However, despite these differences, in this case the personal support and enthusiasm from the supervisor outweighed the academic mismatch to reveal a fruitful and successful relationship.

What type of relationship can I expect?

Once a supervisor has committed to guiding you through the process there is always a 'getting to know you' phase, which will take a few months as you settle into the institution and start to work towards your research design. However, the relationship often starts off laden with expectations on both sides. The supervisor most probably reflects on their own relationship with their supervisor, and also other mentoring relationships and will bring pre-determined expectations to the relationship. Equally, students will no doubt come to the relationship with many expectations and unknowns. Early on a reality check is needed where these expectations are acknowledged and unpacked. Claire Maxwell, who completed a PhD after five years' part-time research, describes the disjuncture between her 'ideal type' and the reality of the supervisory relationship:

> Before I started my PhD I had this fantasy about what it would be like. My supervisor would be this incredible woman, with whom I would form a close bond based on friendship, respect and intellectual stimulation. I envisaged I would spend many an afternoon round her house, sitting on the living room floor drinking cups of tea and putting the world to rights! The reality was quite different.

Managing your own expectations and that of the supervisor is something that needs to be checked from the outset and revisited at different points in the process. In the initial meetings the university regulations should be made clear. These will include what are regarded as the appropriate number of supervision meetings (usually about ten per year) and how these meetings will be conducted. This could include a discussion about work expectations, communication expectations and general ground rules for engagement (see Chapter 15). Again, Claire Maxwell reflects on the importance of re-establishing the parameters of the relationship periodically to take account of new situations:

> At the end of every term or year, I should have had an up-front discussion with my supervisor about how we both felt our supervisor–student relationship was going and discussed any changes we needed to make.

One point that is important to convey about the supervisor–student relationship is that the boundaries of the relationship can often be very different from other relationships you will have previously experienced in education. Bill Armer reflects on the differences between the undergraduate and postgraduate relationship with tutors:

> The relationship between a PhD research student and her/his supervisor(s) is very different to that between taught student and course teacher. The former is a long-term and dynamic thing, the latter fleeting and fixed in its co-ordinates – 'you tutee, me tutor'. In contrast, the PhD student is more of an apprentice than a tutee.

This notion of 'an apprentice' is a worthy analogy. When you start off, the supervisor is the senior expert but it is hoped that in working towards and gaining the PhD the student will come out the other end as an intellectual equal. What will be new in this relationship is how different the parameters and boundaries are compared to other types of formal relationships. The relationship, while being framed by the seriousness of getting the business done, usually takes on an element of personal mentoring, mutual respect and the kind of familiarity that could be considered professional friendship. Bill Armer explains how these elements of a successful personal working relationship can be summarised by the concept 'rapport':

> Supervisors have a need to feel that their student is worthy of respect both professionally and personally. Friendship is not necessary here, but a certain degree of rapport is highly desirable for a working relationship.

So, by now you should have figured out that the relationship with your supervisor is incredibly important but equally of a type that has not been experienced elsewhere. The next bit of news is that it is like the tide: always shifting!

Shifts in the relationship

Like all relationships, that between the supervisor and the student is not static but shifts with time and process. As you become more familiar with each other and the expectations of doing a PhD, the relationship will alter. This is a sign of progress, as Bill Armer suggests:

> The balance of the relationship must shift from that of the naive PhD researcher in need of firm direction and guidance at the beginning. Over time this will ideally change to a passing need for advice and ultimately a mutual discussion between equals.

However, with these changes can occur problems. Many students experience hiccups in what is generally an effective and supportive relationship. This can be because of your own issues, such as a lack of progress, frustration with fieldwork, personal problems or time constraints. Blips that occur in the relationship are often related to miscommunication and unclear expectations, both of which can be sorted out through a specific meeting initiated by you.

BOX 3.3

Bill Armer says: 'Communicate your worries clearly, but also listen carefully to the response. Very often, the problem is simply one of mutual understanding and a "clear the air" meeting is all that is required.'

The supervisor's own career, work commitments and personal circumstances can interfere with your relationship and work trajectory, particularly if they take a sabbatical [study leave], become a visiting fellow elsewhere, or have time off for sickness or maternity/paternity leave. Foreseeable interference regarding supervision should be picked up by the postgraduate tutor, who will put temporary measures in place. Other issues that make you feel dissatisfied with the relationship can usually be ironed out by taking some of the following solutions to short-term problems:

- Call on the postgraduate tutor for independent, confidential advice.
- Seek a second supervisor (temporary or permanent) or rely on the second supervisor if there are problems with the first.
- Proactively find support from others in the department.
- Use supervision through telephone and email contact for a limited period.
- Use your own networks of support.
- Seek further personal support through the counselling service (see Chapter 18).

If your dissatisfaction with the supervisory arrangements is not just a passing phase, or a particular incident has left you feeling wronged, then there are several courses of action available. After all, we are all privy to the horror stories that circulate through the postgraduate networks relating to awful supervision and disruptive relationships that reduce students to gibbering wrecks! If you feel that there is something problematic in the relationship with your supervisor, or feel strongly that you are not getting the support you need, then there are various informal and formal steps that can be taken.

BOX 3.4

The postgraduate tutor is an important mediator, source of independent support, advice and expert knowledge in this role. They should be considered a first port of call before taking issues further and a solution can often be found with their help.

First you must remember that any university is a complex, hierarchical organisation and operates rigid systems, rules and procedures. Where you feel there is a case of negligence or a case for making a formal complaint about an incident, the official route must be taken. University Student Complaints procedures are set down in stone in the regulations (all accessible on the institution's intranet) and further advice should be sought from the Student Union in these matters. There are strict procedures, requirements to submit evidence and stages to the complaints procedure that must be followed. Arming yourself with knowledge of the complaints procedure is a critical starting point.

When your supervisor gets another job

One of the common events that can disrupt a student's PhD progress is their supervisor taking up a wonderful job that they simply couldn't turn down at another university. Sometimes this can be on another continent! Usually the outcomes are not so drastic as academics often negotiate taking their students with them as part of their new work package. This should protect your financial status and maintain your relationship with your supervisor. However, geography can be the biggest upheaval: if your supervisor moves to a neighbouring city then this is not too problematic, but if they relocate further afield then a major decision needs to be made on your part. Students are often given the choice of changing institution and keeping their supervisor, or they are faced with staying put and having a new supervisor.

Sometimes, if funds permit and all are in agreement, the original supervisor can become what is known as a 'long arm' supervisor who will still be involved in your progress and guidance, but your main supervision will be conducted by a new mentor at the original institution where you are registered. This is often the best result as you can then secure continuity of supervision and receive the fresh input of a new supervisor. However, where supervisory relationships become less conventional there is often ground for confusion, limitations on contact and a good relationship potentially turns sour. Claire Maxwell reflects on how, in her second year, her supervisor announced she was taking a career break but would continue her supervisory role. While this seemed only a minor change, Claire felt that in hindsight there was confusion surrounding these new circumstances:

I did not really proactively try to re-negotiate our relationship, so we were both clear what would be expected. Due to this change in circumstances, my university department had to re-assign me a new supervisor, as I needed to have someone responsible for me who worked at the university where I was registered. It took them 18 months to do this!

Given the current emphasis from the Higher Education Agency and the UK Grad Programme on providing effective and consistent supervision and positive postgraduate experiences, we certainly hope that Claire's wait of 18 months for an additional supervisor is a thing of the past. Inevitably, if your supervisor leaves the institution there will be adjustments to make but be assured that other people in the institution, such as the postgraduate tutor, will be looking out for you and offer's an official first port of call.

These issues described above are general characteristics that many supervisor-student relationships experience. However, we also want to acknowledge that there are times when the relationship becomes defunct and something needs to be done about it!

Reasons for changing supervisor

As with all relationships, there may come a time when you consider the dynamics to have reached 'irretrievable breakdown'. There could be a million reasons for this, but what they all lead to is an unworkable relationship that causes you personal distress and intellectual stagnation. Christine Rogers notes that there can be intractable difficulties if the ages of the supervisor and student are similar and there is an authoritarian streak to the mentoring:

My supervisor was only a few years older than me and made me feel like I was inferior. She told me what to do and said that I should use her experience. I'm afraid this way of working brought out the rebel in me.

The rapport that we previously mentioned as a key ingredient to a relationship simply may not be there and, as in all walks of life, there can be a clash of styles and personalities. Where you feel the relationship is simply not working after you have made a considerable effort, then it is time to think about approaching the postgraduate tutor to discuss changing your supervisor. However, this may be easier said than done. Bill Armer reflects on how, despite both parties amicably agreeing that the relationship was not productive and that a change of supervisor was needed, the official procedures took time and negotiation to fulfil:

I found that my supervisor could only withdraw by claiming that I was failing to progress in a satisfactory manner, whilst I had, as it were, to petition for divorce on the grounds of an 'irretrievable breakdown' in the relationship.

If you feel that the relationship is tainted with unprofessional conduct on the part of the supervisor then this is a clear reason to seek change and possibly take the matter further. Prejudicial attitudes, practices and behaviours should be taken up through formal routes. In cases where romantic relationships develop between the student and supervisor the university's code of conduct should be consulted on these matters. There are inherent power issues here due to the academic holding a supervisory role, which means that mentoring usually cannot continue because of a conflict of personal interest.

Realising that you are in the wrong relationship may not be a result of any personal incompatibility, but a wider realisation of what you want out of the PhD. Nicola Scott's case is an interesting reflection on how the root of the discontent may be that you are in the wrong discipline or department. Nicola studied politics up to masters level before winning a scholarship in social anthropology, which was a new discipline for her. She explains what happened:

Despite the fact that my supervisor and department were excellent, throughout my first year I began to feel isolated from my peers. Consequently, I began to lose self-confidence in my ability to do a PhD. Feeling privileged to be a scholarship holder and looking forward to conducting overseas fieldwork, the passion for my topic prevented me from deserting my studies. Once I was abroad I had time to think about what I wanted from my PhD and realised I could not continue unless I could return to the discipline I felt most comfortable with. I informed my supervisor and was very open and honest about my preference to discontinue with anthropology. My supervisor was very understanding and I made a case to transfer my funding to another department where I found a new supervisor. I only wish I had informed my first supervisor much sooner about my wish to transfer rather than spend a year worrying about the discipline within which my PhD was located.

Feeling 'at home' with a discipline is as important as making the right decisions about who will be your mentor and whether you can do business together. Nicola's scenario highlights that recognising there is a problem early on and seeking advice can save much angst and time. If you want to make changes do not think that you will be the first person to do so – these changes are much more common than you think.

Finding a new mentor

Where both parties are happy with a change of supervisory arrangements, finding a new supervisor within the department can work fairly informally. Christine Rogers explains how she decided to leave her original supervisor, who was chosen because of an already established supervisory relationship at undergraduate level, for someone who was working within an area closer to her own research area:

My original supervisor was understanding and thought the change was good, as we had worked together before. There was no animosity as the reasons for 'leaving' him were not a reflection on him but a desire to work with someone who had some research experience in education.

Speaking to the relevant people, completing the paperwork and checking with the funding body are the minimum requirements for making a change. Prepare for delays. Finding a new mentor when academics are often over-burdened with duties and students is not necessarily easy. Remember though the department also has a responsibility to ensure you have adequate supervision, as with most solutions for difficulties with the PhD being proactive in recruiting a new supervisor is the best step forward. Seeking out a new mentor rather than relying on allocation is particularly important second time round because you want to make sure that the questions you did not ask initially are not only asked this time but you will also be better placed to know if the answers are acceptable to you. Don't be surprised if there are also internal politics that you have to manage, including dismantling some stereotypes about being a 'troublemaker'. When scouting the department for a new mentor Bill Armer was concerned that he was perceived as 'damaged goods' by prospective supervisors:

> Without being officially declared an untouchable, it was amazing how many members of the Faculty had a full workload already, had study leave scheduled for next year or did not feel that my research topic fell within their area. This does little for one's self-esteem!

It should not be under-estimated how difficult any phase of unsettlement may be when changing supervisor, finding a new one and starting the process all over again. It is quite normal at this time to feel vulnerable, inadequate, low in confidence and frustrated at a situation that you feel is out of your hands. Often taking a few weeks out to reflect, get advice and make some positive decisions is a productive exercise. After all, nothing worthwhile can be written while the infrastructure of your PhD is shaky. However, this unsettled phase should only be short term, as between your own motivation to change, proactively seeking an alternative mentor and the university system recognising there is a problem, solutions should be found before your work is significantly affected.

BOX 3.5

It is as much for you to actively interview a prospective supervisor as *vice-versa*.

Key Points to Remember

▶ Whether you approach an academic or you are allocated a supervisor, consider whether you can 'do business' with this person.

▶ The student–supervisor relationship is unique, often based on informalities yet framed in a hierarchical and bureaucratic system.

- ► Expect the relationship to shift as you progress and be prepared to re-negotiate expectations.
- ► Supervisors can move institutions, leaving you with some difficult decisions to make.
- ► Make regular contact with other sources of support in the department, particularly the postgraduate tutor.
- ► Dissatisfaction with the supervisory arrangements can often be sorted out amicably and informally.
- ► Where more serious issues of unprofessional conduct occur then the University complaints procedure is the best option.
- ► Be guided by the rules and procedures – universities are big old bureaucracies.
- ► When finding a new supervisor make sure you go over all the questions you now know you should have asked before!

SUGGESTED READING

Cryer, P. (2006) *The Research Student's Guide to Success,* 3rd edn. Maidenhead: Open University Press. Chapter 6 'Interacting with Supervisors'.

Eley, A.R. and Jennings, R. (2005) *Effective Postgraduate Supervision: Improving the Student/Supervisor Relationship.* Maidenhead: Open University Press.

Marshall, S. and Green, N. (2004) *Your PhD Companion.* Oxford: How To Books. Chapter 3 'You and Your Supervisor'.

Rugg, G. and Petre, M. (2004) *The Unwritten Rules of PhD Research.* Maidenhead: Open University Press.

Chapter 4
Managing the Ethics of Academia

Why bother with ethics?

All research conducted, whether in the natural sciences or social sciences and humanities, involves ethical issues to a lesser or greater degree. It has been argued that all knowledge production has ethical implications (Miller and Bell, 2002) and therefore will be of concern to all postgraduates. Primarily this is because, as researchers, we are engaging with the social world and human beings to access information and inquire into people's lives and experiences. Ethics, ethical dilemmas and the responsibilities of researchers to produce ethical knowledge have increasingly been written about, with the number of publications and student resources growing in this area. All of the academic disciplines have their own historical development of ethical practice, as ethics is not only about 'doing' good research, but protecting the reputation and maintaining high research standards for the individual researcher, the discipline and the wider research community. There has been much talk in social sciences about the 'ethical turn' whereby the process of ethics, monitoring research and surveying what researchers are doing has created a bureaucracy of ethical governance which has both negative and positive implications for the quality of data (Crow et al., 2006). There are many dimensions of 'ethics in research' to the extent that students first exploring ethical issues in their own studies are often overwhelmed by the enormity of the literature out there and the potentially vast number of issues to consider. Teela Sanders found that in her musings over ethics and ethical governance in academia (researching in the sex industry, ethics has been a preoccupation for some years), it is useful to examine ethics in three separate ways.

1   Ethics as an intellectual subject that raises important and interesting questions about the nature of interacting with respondents. Being ethical can involve enhancing research 'reflexivity' (reflecting on the role of the researcher in the relationship with their research 'subjects', the fieldwork setting and the creation of knowledge). In addition, ethical dilemmas and decision making raise wider philosophical questions about the nature and production of knowledge, its validity and reliability. For instance, Le Voi (2002: 155) makes the direct point that 'faking research is a case of fraud against the whole process of research'.

2   Ethical practice can be considered in relation to responsibilities and rights. Good practice in research has concepts such as respect and beneficence as core principles of research procedures. Individuals have the right not to be introduced to harm (whether physical, emotional or psychological); there are rights around privacy, confidentiality, anonymity and informed consent. It is the researcher's responsibility (and also that of the institution) to carry out ethically sound social inquiry that does not harm anyone. Equally, as a researcher, your own rights need to be considered in relation to potential harms and safety issues.

3   Ethics can be considered in terms of the procedural expectations of doing research in a university setting. There is a whole bureaucracy around ethics in the form of Research Ethics Committees, internal processes such as ethics panels and forms to fill in for that final seal of approval before the project begins. The procedural expectations around ethics flag up legal issues in relation to legislation such as the Data Protection Act, 1984, and the Freedom of Information Act, 2000. Beyond these procedures though, ethics needs to be considered and reviewed throughout the life of a research project.

BOX 4.1   Ethical governance

What has come to be known as ethical governance of the research industry is having an impact on the processes of approval before research can get under way. This will filter down to postgraduates who will have to justify that their project is ethical in formal ways, according to official criteria.

As you can see, there is a lot to think about. But don't get despondent. Seek out the increasing number of textbooks, seminars or university courses on research ethics that will help you clarify the specific issues you need to consider. This chapter acts as an introduction to some key areas to think about when you are planning your research project.

Doing ethical research

The ethical issues that you will need to think about, plan for and design your research around will be specific to your own study. The ethical dimensions will be determined by what your research questions are and, if you are doing fieldwork, then ethical issues will arise from with whom, what and where fieldwork takes place. Doing ethical research is also about taking part in a wider research community and upholding academic integrity. The research community that you are representing and involved with as a postgraduate student is based on a set of principles that supports its reputation as a responsible profession. Within this there are criteria on which the quality of research is judged and a set of expectations about 'good' and 'bad' research methodology and design. Credibility is only given to research findings and projects that stay within the ethical guidelines and uphold the integrity of the research community by promoting and practising ethically sound research.

Within these broader aims of maintaining (and indeed gaining for yourself) academic integrity, there are some standard criteria you need to cover when conducting empirical studies that involve collecting information from individuals or doing secondary data analysis. The key criteria, which you may remember from undergraduate methods courses, are informed consent, confidentiality and anonymity.

BOX 4.2   Ethics as part of the data

'I learned a great deal about my research from the ethical decisions that I was required to make. They can reveal so much in terms of power relations in the research context – we often forget that this is part of the fieldwork itself. Rather than treating these issues as problems, they should be seen as obstacles that can provide their own rich source of data.'

[Kate Williams]

The process of informed consent

In the Appendix you will find an example of an informed consent form and an information sheet for respondents that Sharon Elley used when researching young people's experiences. These forms are examples of one type of procedure when asking someone to take part in your research. The information sheet has specific details of the project, such as the aims and objectives, who is associated with the research and what will be required from the respondent. The informed consent form is the part where permission is asked from the individual about their understanding of the project, what is expected of them, their rights and their voluntary participation.

Gaining consent from people to be included in the research has been described as a process and not a form. Sharon spent time at the beginning of the interview going through the information sheet and explaining further any issues that were not clear and taking questions from the young person. In addition, because the respondent was under 18, she specifically wanted to gain written consent. However, it was important not just to give the consent form to the young person to read and sign, but to go through the details of the consent form and make sure the respondent was clear about what they were signing up for. Any further participation would also require re-negotiation of any consent to take part, with the respondent having the right not to participate further at any stage.

The process of informed consent needs to be thought about in relation to the specific characteristics and context of your project. Informed consent can be gained in other ways, not just through a signed form. For instance, when Teela Sanders researched sex workers she verbally explained the aims and objectives of the research, what would be done with the findings and how the respondents' verbatim comments would be used. She also set out what would be done with the transcripts and tapes after the project had finished. Consent to participate in the study was then obtained verbally with no additional consent form to sign. This was partly because of the practicalities of the places where the sex workers were interviewed, and also because the sex workers often wanted to keep their identity completely secret (even from their colleagues and the researcher), so they did not want their signature on a piece of paper (see Sanders, 2005, 2006 for more details).

The principles and procedures surrounding informed consent have been hotly debated, mainly questioning what it is that participants are consenting to (Miller and Bell, 2002). There are also limitations to gaining informed consent because respondents need to be able to understand what they are fully consenting to. For instance, Coomber (2002) notes the limitations of gaining written consent in the case of studying people with criminal convictions. Also, it may be the case that the full extent or details of the specific research questions are not revealed to the respondents.

Despite the contentious nature of informed consent, the basic issue is that the respondents are taking part in the research on a voluntary basis. Whatever format informed consent takes in your project, you need to consider the following points:

- What are you asking for?
- How will you explain the research questions to the respondent?
- How much is the consent process part of trust and rapport building?
- What will you do with the data, who will listen to the recordings or see the transcripts?
- Where will you store the information?
- What support is in place for potential 'fallout' from interview?
- How can you ensure confidentiality and anonymity, and harm-free research?
- Are there communication barriers (language, capacity to understand, requirements for people living with impairments)?

There has been some recent criticism about the over-zealous expectations around gaining consent from people which can result in the ethics of the project overriding the process of establishing trust and collecting data. Crow et al. (2006) note from research findings that the production of data, and certainly good quality data, can be hindered by an over-emphasis on informed consent. For instance, practical arrangements for getting a form signed can override the relationship building that researchers must do to gain rapport, and therefore can reduce participation rates. This highlights how approaches to ethical practice affect the relationship between the researcher and the respondent and may have an influence on the process of data collection and subsequent findings.

Confidentiality and anonymity

The rights of respondents to confidentiality are at the core of the responsibilities and obligations of the researcher. Individual privacy needs to be respected and this has significant implications for how the data is collected, analysed, stored, reported and disseminated. Remember that a thesis is a public document and that anything written for publication is accessible to the public. Therefore confidentiality is a key point to consider, particularly when reporting findings and disseminating information through the media for example. Also, in the information sheet (see Appendix 2), details should be offered about where the information will be stored and who will have access to the transcripts and tapes. Safe and secure storage is also a part of maintaining ethical practice and should be considered before you have finished the project (see Chapter 5).

Most cases of protecting anonymity are straightforward as respondents do not want to be identified and there are standard processes for de-identifying individuals so that the data cannot be traced back to them. However, anonymity is not just about the individual that gave the information as other people and places can be identified in the research. Findings may identify a town or city, an organisation or group, a place or building, as well as individuals who are mentioned directly in the research. Becky Tipper recalls how the issue of anonymity became a stumbling block in her research with young children as unexpected dynamics between the respondents and the purpose of the research brought into question the role of anonymised interviews:

> Power relations are certainly important, but in subtle and surprising ways, and children are far from simply passive and vulnerable research subjects. For instance, conventionally in qualitative data all names and places are anonymised. However, several children have asked for their *real* names to be used in publications. There is a strong rationale for anonymisation, since it protects *other* people discussed in interviews. Nevertheless, this project is designed explicitly to give children a 'voice' in an adult-focused society, and children have been keen to participate for *precisely this reason*. Having promised them a chance to present *their* perspectives, am I hypocritical to insist that their names are anonymised?

Research is often about topics that are current to local and national communities and can involve highly sensitive and controversial topics. Kate Williams was investigating the community relationships that surrounded the rise of a resident action group to resist street prostitution in a local neighbourhood. Kate recounts how assuring confidentiality was not straightforward:

Applying anonymity invariably places the researcher in a position of significant responsibility as it is very difficult to guarantee. I made every attempt to secure anonymity for my respondents, but felt uncomfortable as my fieldwork site and the research area that I was covering had not only been very high profile in the region but had also received a great deal of press attention nationally. Due to the controversial nature of the research, I was only too aware that for certain key respondents, being identified could potentially lead to real personal or professional threats and dangers.

Often ethical issues raise many more questions than answers! After all they often entail moral and philosophical dilemmas that do not have obvious outcomes or solutions. Even if your project is fairly conventional you will make decisions about what anonymisation process you will adopt. For instance, will the data be anonymised at the point of collection or transcription or be left until the analysis stage? When anonymisation is completed how will you identify the respondents – by pseudonyms, numbers, or stating key socio-demographic characteristics? A stage dedicated to anonymising data will be required in your timetable.

BOX 4.3   Do no harm

All researchers have a 'Duty of Care' not to introduce any additional harm into participants' lives. Maintaining respect, integrity and conducting research with strong regard for moral and legal rights are the minimum expectations.

In some cases it may be appropriate to modify conventional practices. As there are limitations with informed consent, confidentiality also has its limitations, and in specific cases it is the researcher's responsibility to break confidentiality, in the context of other over-riding ethical concerns such as in relation to the safety of young people. This is usually the case where the researcher is concerned that the respondent is at risk of harm or has disclosed information of harm. The limits to confidentiality must be set out in the informed consent stage (see the form in the Appendix) and if incidents like this occur then seek support from supervisors or an ethics panel at university. This highlights the limits of confidentiality but also how researchers are accountable to a range of audiences and that research is not conducted in a bubble but is a real life activity.

One size does not fit all

Although there are basic criteria that are required by the academic community and indeed Research Ethics Committees, there are always complications, exceptions and dilemmas in ethical decision making. Different research groups present different ethical issues. For instance, if you are researching vulnerable adults who are marginalised from society, there are issues about exploitation and 'taking information' from respondents who are relatively powerless in relation to material, social and intellectual resources. Even at the dissemination stage, careful thought needs to be given to the potential impact of findings on research participants, who can suffer further marginalisation (and different issues may need thinking through when doing research with 'elites'). If you are researching certain groups in settings that affect their freedom and rights, such as a prison or a hospital, there are other conditions to consider. Becky Tipper was doing her PhD part-time whilst working on a research project. She reflects on how ethical issues were at the forefront of her thinking when she started the project because her sample group were young children. The age of the group of respondents raised particular issues in relation to consent and power:

When I started out on this research project with children aged 7–11, it seemed that the ethical concerns would be particularly complex. Was it really possible to obtain 'informed consent' from children? Could I be sure they fully understood what was involved? What would I do if children revealed information about abuse or harm? How could I minimise the potential imbalance of power and verbal articulacy in interviews between young children and myself – an adult academic researcher? It seemed that I would be navigating a practical and ethical minefield!

Different research methods that are applied in a project present different ethical issues. Although the standard criteria described above are present in most of the methods that span the qualitative and quantitative divide, different methods will raise a variety of ethical issues. For example, doing covert research (which is usually associated with ethnography and observations) is always considered an ethical sticking point because of the centrality of informed consent and also the right to voluntary participation. Yet there may be certain circumstances where covert research is justifiable as there are no other ways to gain access to certain groups or activities without having a significant impact on the group behaviour. Ethnographic methods, especially observation, can present the researcher with some serious dilemmas that were not necessarily considered during the research design stage. Reflecting on her own research with female sex workers in brothels and massage parlours, Teela Sanders recalls ethical dilemmas around observing what happens in sex work venues. Her success at building up co-operative relationships with informants presented new ethical dilemmas:

> When Astrid, an experienced sex worker with whom I had sat for many hours, invited me into the room to 'see how clinical it was', I should not have been shocked but perhaps delighted at the chance to move from the periphery where I lurked to the centre as an insider. After all, I grappled, isn't this the ultimate objective of the participant observer? I had to weigh up why watching the sexual interaction was so different to watching other aspects of the commercial transaction and how observing sex would alter the parameters of the research? (Sanders, 2005: 209)

Researching those who are considered relatively powerless is not the only instance that warrants specific ethical consideration. Elites, such as multi-national company directors, and those who may be identifiable by their job titles also need to be protected. With ethnographic methods much of the 'ethical stuff' cannot be pre-empted, so must be dealt with *in situ*, when you are there in the field, in the thick of the action. Referring to the framework of rights and responsibilities usually provides the answer to tricky situations, but you may have to work some solutions out for yourself.

BOX 4.5   Accountability

As researchers we are accountable to a range of audiences and each demand their own ethical consideration. Think about accountability as a researcher to the following groups:

- Your institution
- Your supervisor
- Your informants
- Your gatekeepers
- The wider research community
- Yourself

The role of research ethics committees

Traditionally, doctoral students have always discussed ethical issues with their supervisor and at upgrade assessments to monitor what issues may arise and how they should be handled. Now ethics have become a central part of the research process in universities and research communities. When applying for funding, ethical approval must be sought and usually passed through an internal panel called a Research Ethics Committee. These are bureaucratic systems of checking that a researcher has the legal issues covered, has designed appropriate ethical methodology and has considered the setting and what specific risks may occur. In part, this is like a risk assessment for respondents and the researcher, but it is also about the reputation and integrity of the university. Living in a world of litigation, ethics is becoming an important issue for university lawyers. There has been much criticism of the introduction of bureaucracy and checking systems around ethics, mainly because social science has traditionally been very good at performing ethically sound research as there are substantive discipline guidelines. At worst, criticism suggests that ethics committees, apart from taking a huge amount of time and effort, are policing research methods and topics rather than just looking at ethical issues. This means that ethics committees could squeeze out innovative research or risky topics and populations as they are considered too problematic.

Research ethics committees essentially reinforce the guidelines that each discipline has worked by for some time. The Social Research Association, established in 1978, produced the *Respect Code of Practice for Socio-Economic Research* (www.the-sra. org.uk/ethicals/htm). This Code acts as 'a voluntary code of practice covering the conduct of socio-economic research in Europe' which promotes three underlying principles:

- Upholding scientific standards.
- Compliance with law.
- Avoidance of social and personal harm.

Codes of practice for various social science and humanities disciplines are available from relevant professional bodies and associations that represent the discipline. For instance, the following organisations have useful codes of ethical practice:

- British Psychological Society: www.bps.org.uk
- Social Policy Association: www.social-policy.com
- British Sociological Association: www.britsoc.co.uk
- British Educational Research Association: http://www.bera.ac.uk/
- British Society of Criminology: www.britsoccrim.org/ethical.htm

The types of issues and complexities of ethics that all researchers need to consider can be understood by the breadth of coverage in the Statement of Ethical Practice for the British Sociological Association. This code covers the following areas:

- Professional integrity.
- Relations with and responsibilities towards research participants.
- Relationships with research participants.
- Covert research.
- Anonymity, privacy and confidentiality.
- Relations with and responsibilities towards sponsors.
- Clarifying obligations, roles and rights.
- Pre-empting outcomes and negotiations about research.
- Obligations to sponsors and funders during the research process.

As previously mentioned, researchers have legal responsibilities in relation to collecting, storing and protecting data (see Box 4.6).

BOX 4.6   Research responsibilities for data protection

All researchers need to uphold their legal responsibilities for data protection. Conventions among social science researchers include the following strategies for anonymising and ethically storing personal information:

1   The act of collecting personal data needs to have a research rationale that is clearly explained to any research participant.
2   Seek informed consent via explaining the rationale behind information collecting and gaining permission to collect the data. Respondents reserve the right to decline this request.
3   Asking about income, education, occupation or family details requires ethical considerations as many may feel these issues are personal and private. Think about how you ask for this information and your information needs. Will asking respondent to tick an income range (i.e. £10,000–15,000 pa), education range or general occupation category suffice?
4   Make a log, chart, file or some sort of master sheet of all the personal details about each research respondent and research settings. Attach an anonymous label to each data case and setting.
5   Anonymise all personal information throughout your data cases both in the body of the data and the respondent details.
6   Make sure the log of personal details is only accessible to you or additional colleagues working on the research project. All personal information needs to be securely stored, i.e. on a separate PC file that is password protected, or in a locked drawer/filing cabinet.
7   Seek to protect the respondent's integrity and anonymous status throughout data analysis and writing up.

Personal ethics in research practice

A lot of the emphasis in designing ethical research is on the safety and rights of the respondent, ensuring that they come to no harm. However, the safety of the researcher is also an important consideration across the research project such as when accessing research participants, dealing with gatekeepers or conducting fieldwork. The complex nature of 'risk' in research has been documented more frequently recently, as often the risks are unforeseen and develop *in situ* when the research is taking place in the field (Lee-Treweek and Linkogle, 2000). The personal impact of research, especially fieldwork, must be taken into consideration. You may need to think about your safety and think about whether you are going to places that may be risky or put you in danger. Emotional danger and emotions in research also need to be given consideration. For instance, Sharon Elley recalls how her interview work with young people about sex education programmes could involve emotionally and ethically challenging interactions:

I vividly recall an interview where a seventeen-year-old disclosed rape at the age of ten. Emotionally I felt stunned and horrified; professionally I felt ill-equipped to deal with the moment. Ethically, I'd accounted for this but I was unsure of what to do next. Ethical and professional guidelines flooded my mind as I asked myself 'What am I supposed to do now?' Do I ask her if she wants to discuss it; do I skirt around it; can I deal with what she reveals? Notwithstanding, we have a 'Duty of Care', responsibilities and obligations towards young people. So, tentatively I asked her if she wanted to talk about it and she replied 'No'. The interview continued but I felt subdued and there was a crawling in my stomach. Afterwards, I passed the information on to the appropriate persons but I questioned whether in doing so I was making the young woman relive past experiences again in order to tick the appropriate boxes. Yet still I realise such procedures need to be in place to protect others.

This highlights how there are ethical dilemmas that have to be confronted on the spot in the field and dealt with as a real life issue and not just a potential consideration in a research design paper. The ethical decisions have impacts on individuals and good accounts of 'tales in the field' offer glimpses into what it is actually like to do research. As researchers the personal and safety issues in relation to our fieldwork are key consideration. Kate Williams recounts fear in the fieldwork process and highlights that safety procedures should be paramount to protect yourself from harm:

> As a female I felt particularly vulnerable when visiting people's houses alone to conduct interviews, and always left appropriate details with a member of my family. Nonetheless, situations still occurred that caused me to feel threatened. For example, I had to use my judgement on whether to continue when a sex worker that I was interviewing told me that her violent pimp could return at any time. Although I stayed on that occasion, I did turn down other potential fieldwork opportunities due to personal safety fears. As much as we want the data, we have to do everything possible to protect ourselves.

Ethics are important in research and as a student you will encounter them both professionally and personally. In an age of ethical governance where research can be constrained by the bureaucracy around checking what we are doing is legitimate, as a student you will have ethics at the forefront of your thinking, planning and real life experience in the field.

Key Points to Remember

▶ Good practice will be a guiding principle of your research.
▶ You will probably have to go through a formal ethics committee at university.
▶ The main issues to consider are potential harms, confidentiality and informed consent.
▶ Researching vulnerable groups will pose specific ethical issues.
▶ Certain methodologies, such as ethnography, may prove more complicated than other methods, but do not be deterred.
▶ It is important to think about your own safety.
▶ Ethical issues cannot always be second-guessed – be prepared for the unexpected and to make decisions in the field.
▶ Your discipline will have a useful code of practice to follow.
▶ Part of your research training should include investigation of ethical standards and approaches within your field of research.

SUGGESTED READING

Denscombe, M. (2002) *Ground Rules for Good Research*: *A 10 Point Guide for Social Researchers*. Buckingham: Open University Press.

Le Voi, M. (2002) 'Responsibilities, rights and ethics', in S. Potter (ed.), *Doing Postgraduate Research.* London: Open University and Sage Publications. pp. 133–153.

Mauthner, M., Birch, M., Jessop, J. and Miller, T. (eds) (2002) *Ethics in Qualitative Research*. London: Sage.

Oliver, P. (2003) *The Student's Guide to Research Ethics*. Maidenhead: Open University Press.

Chapter 5
What to do With your Data

From data to findings

A clear distinction between data collection and data analysis is difficult to maintain as researchers can begin to interpret data as it is collected (hopefully capturing such hunches and impressions in a research diary or log). However, data analysis refers to a more concentrated and systematic period of analysing of your data, with the view to generating avenues for further data collection or your overall research findings. The process of data analysis involves making sense of your data in relation to your research questions. Before considering some important stages and approaches, we need to distinguish between types of data.

Types of data and data analysis
Data can be:

- Numerical (e.g. numbers and measurements).
- Textual (e.g. in written form such as documents; transcripts of individual or group interviews; observational field notes; diary entries or historical records).
- Visual (e.g. such as video recordings; photos).
- Audio (e.g. sound recordings; recorded conversations).
- A mixture of any of the above.

These different types of data offer different ways of capturing the phenomena you are investigating. They can be grouped into quantitative or qualitative forms of data, with the former involving the generation of numerical data and the latter involving interpretations using words, pictures or sounds. Data analysis approaches also involve quantitative, qualitative or combined frameworks.

BOX 5.1   Examples of quantitative and qualitative approaches

Quantitative analysis can involve the production of:

- Descriptive statistics on your data (i.e. variable frequency/averages).
- Inferential statistics (i.e. variable significance/association significance).
- Multivariate analysis (i.e. relationships between two or more variables).

Qualitative analysis also takes many forms including:

- Interpretative thematic data analysis: generating themes from interview, visual or audio data.
- Framework analysis: a thematic approach that seeks to generate concepts from data and a prior evidence base for applied policy research.
- Grounded theory: an approach to generating conceptual frameworks from your data rather than prior academic theory.
- Life story approaches: analysing personal narratives and life stories using theories and biographical frameworks.
- Analysing biography and social context: Biographical Narrative Interpretative Method, for example, seeks to generate a picture of life histories and social contexts.
- Reflexive readings: autobiographical approaches seek to analyse the researcher's life experiences or input into the research process.

At the design phase of your study, we are hoping that you have already considered your analytical approach and established a complementary connection between your research questions, data collection and analysis methods and approach. Box 5.1 also gives some further indications of approaches on which the suggested reading at the end of this chapter provides more information (also see Chapter 2). Not having a clear plan of how you propose to analyse your data runs the risk of being limited in the kind of analysis you can do. Planning your analysis approach after data collection increases the likelihood of being restricted to the kinds of analysis that suit the data you have collected. For example, a qualitative researcher is unable to conduct a biographical life history approach to analysis if they have limited data on the respondent's life history; and a quantitative researcher will find it difficult to conduct particular types of statistical analysis of their data if their questions or sampling method do not fit the analysis approach. However, with many existing texts that detail particular approaches, this chapter tends to refer students on to more specialist texts for more detailed accounts and here considers some steps and strategies for moving through your analysis in a more general way. The chapter begins with some experiential reflections on getting started and then goes on to consider issues for analysis such as planning your approach, preparing your data, indexing and coding, and establishing relationships, patterns and findings.

Getting started, getting stuck and pushing forward

Undertaking a PhD study will inevitably involve periods of uncertainty, difficulty and doubt. A common sentiment at the beginning of the data analysis stage is an overwhelming feeling of having a lot of data and wondering what to do with it, and whether it will provide some illuminating answers to your questions. One of our contributors, Joseph Burridge, undertook a study of media representations of Iraq. He was all set to begin his PhD research at the end of September 2001 when the World Trade Centre was struck earlier that month. This event changed the significance of his project. Joseph then spent three years collecting a huge amount of newspaper archive data:

> My data collection began a fortnight before the official start of my PhD registration (12th September 2001), and continued up until about a fortnight before my thesis was submitted. The availability of masses of material can be viewed as either extremely exciting or as potentially overwhelming – I constantly oscillated between these two positions. In reality, I spent several hours each day collating and categorising media reports.

Several of our contributors found that they had under-estimated the time it would take to analyse the data they collected. Harriet Churchill realised she had collected more qualitative interview data than she was able to analyse, which contributed to a delay in submission by six months. Due to time constraints, John Roberts decided to drop an area of historical data archive material in his project, but was able to return to analyse this at a later date. Often the time taken to 'prepare' your data for analysis such as with inputting data into software programs, can be grossly under-estimated. Emily Tanner felt she had:

> Under-estimated the amount of time it would take to prepare the (quantitative) data for analysis. It took much more time than expected to spot the errors in data entry to SPSS, to deal with missing data and to derive the variable for subsequent analysis.

Another concern in the early stages of data analysis was one of doubt and uncertainty over whether 'you have the right data or will find anything out'. This can sometimes be even more the case in survey research, as you may not have read through your survey responses until you begin analysis. In her quantitative study of maternal employment outcomes, Emily Tanner was concerned about 'whether I would find the relationships that I was expecting or if my results will yield anything to write about'. With no scope to further probe your participants' responses in postal survey research, Sheelah Flatman Watson was hugely concerned whether her 'questions were right' or understood appropriately. She waited with 'nervous anticipation' for her surveys to be returned and to find out if 'her questions were appropriate, and if there was enough scope for individual comment in the open questions' she had devised.

A further common challenge within the data analysis phase of a research project is that of moving from a detailed picture of your data, perhaps aided by coding, sorting and devising charts and tables of your overall data, towards some overall general explanations and findings. Harriet Churchill discusses this stage of her thematic qualitative data analysis:

> Trying to make connections across all the transcripts was extremely difficult. I found it hard to move towards a more general picture as there seemed to be exceptions to each overall explanation. It wasn't until I started writing up, writing papers and trying to explain the dominant themes in writing that I began to move towards a more general picture of the data. I also had to drop many interesting themes, and really focus on some particularly pertinent areas. Here I was concerned about prematurely limiting my explanatory possibilities.

In moving from data collection towards data analysis you may feel:

- Unsure if you have 'enough' of the 'right' data.
- Unsure if you have 'too much' data.

- Uncertain about how to get 'started'.
- Excited to establish the central findings from the data.
- Unsure about the details of how to put your approach into practice.
- Overwhelmed by the need to learn new data analysis software packages.

To get yourself started with data analysis, it may be worth spending some time reflecting on what your concerns are and what you are expecting to find out, and turning these into questions and issues to think about further and seek advice on. Whether studies employ a qualitative, quantitative or mixed methods approach; analysis requires preparing the data for analysis, employing analytical strategies and moving towards research findings.

Preparing data for analysis

There are a number of tasks involved in preparing your data for further analysis. Data will need to be organised, labelled and stored in ways that are suitable to your purpose and approach. For qualitative data, preparing your data may involve typing up field notes, transcribing interviews, anonymising data and inputting data into a software package. For quantitative data, also you will need to input data into a software package alongside the cataloguing of survey responses, survey response rates and missing data (numerically cataloguing how many surveys responses were received and how many questions were answered in the appropriate way). As we have already highlighted, the time required for these activities, which often overlap between data collection and data analysis, is often under-estimated. However, ultimately thorough and thoughtful preparation of your data will potentially save you some stress and time later on, as you will be able to manage your data in an efficient way. We will now turn to consider four key aspects of data preparation: transcribing qualitative data; labelling and storing data; utilising software packages and preparing quantitative data for analysis. All four of these activities may be carried out as you collect your data and further as a distinctive pre-data analysis stage in your research project.

Preparing data transcripts and field notes
Transcribing a research interview or recorded field notes generates a typed verbatim transcript of the interview or observed interactions and activities. This can help the researcher to analyse interview or observational data in some depth. However, in some studies time constraints may mean that interviews or field conversations are purposefully more partially transcribed, selectively recording data that is deemed to be particularly relevant to the research topic and questions. Alternatively there are very detailed approaches to the transcription of qualitative data that seek to record a vast array of non-verbal and detailed verbal communication. Your transcription approach will really depend on what type of analysis you wish to pursue, your timescale and the resources available.

Italics or **bold** or <u>underline</u> = emphasises a word

(...) = pauses

= for simultaneous speech

CAPS = loud sounding words

(??) = words that the transcriber cannot hear

/ = a rising intonation

full stops, commas and paragraphs at points that seem to indicate these kinds of pauses and endings.

As you type out your interview be generous with your spacing and layout to leave room to write in notes/label segments of text.

Labelling, record keeping, storing and archiving

Good practice here may be to devise a 'data record sheet' for each interview, field visit, survey participant or archived raw data; and to do this before you collect any data so that the details can be filled in as your data comes in. This sheet can include personal details, the date that data was collected, an anonymous code referring to each participant or case and immediate impressions. Alternatively the details can be recorded during data collection in note form and transferred onto a data record sheet in these preliminary stages of data analysis (see Chapter 3 for researcher responsibilities).

Joseph Burridge found it took some time to devise an appropriate system of storing newspaper reports for his study. He ended up devising a manual archiving system, with newspaper reports filed according to a thematic main story approach. Alternatively a number of software packages now exist – although we cannot strongly enough recommend that regular printed out hard copies and back up files of all data files are also securely kept throughout the data analysis phase.

Shall I use a software program?

There are many software programs designed to aid quantitative and qualitative data organisation and analysis. An example of a quantitative program is SPSS (Statistical Package for the Social Sciences) and qualitative ones (called Computer Assisted Qualitative Data Analysis Systems – CAQDAS) are packages such as Atlas.ti, NUD*IST, NVivo 7, Ethnograph and Hypersoft. SPSS is used for the manipulation of numerical data and can compute a number of descriptive, inferential and multivariate statistical tests. CAQDAS can offer a range of indexing, retrieval, organising and note-taking facilities that can be used by a researcher to enhance their data organisation and analysis. Both quantitative and qualitative packages are aids to cataloguing, storing and analysing large amounts of data that would be much more time-consuming and cumbersome to work with manually. SPSS offers massive scope in computing statistical formulae across large data sets in a matter of seconds. CAQDAS also offer more efficient and accessible ways of retrieving and storing qualitative data, as well as offering hyperlink facilities so that different sections of data within or across transcripts or even across different types of data such as photos, video clips, background research notes and field notes can be linked within the program. If these questions appear to be bewildering, you may need to spend some time familiarising yourself with the software packages available for your data analysis purposes. It is common for students to need to supplement their research methods training with more specialist training in particular software packages. Again this requires time and effort. Sheelah Flatman Watson offers an encouraging example of taking the opportunity to enhance her professional development as a researcher when she took on to learn how to use SPSS and NUD*IST6 during her mixed method research study:

> My computer skills were limited. I had a very basic understanding of SPSS. I knew what the package had potential to do having attended a methods class, but I had never applied the learning. My first supervisor was not familiar with SPSS but at least my second supervisor, an SPSS user, helped with how to set up my data. But mainly I had to learn quickly, and decide on an appropriate coding frame. This required hours of trial and error.

BOX 5.3 The use of SPSS and CAQDAS needs to be researcher and methodologically driven

Software programs do not do your analysis for you but operate a number of pre-programmed functions that can support your analysis in particular ways. You will need to have a clear and appropriate rationale for utilising a program and its functions and be aware of the possibilities and limitations built into it. For those using SPSS, familiarity with the rationales underpinning a variety of statistical tests is required as is careful inputting of data in order to make sure the raw data is correct before the software conducts any tests. The different CAQDAS available are underpinned by different explanatory logics. In considering the use of software for your analysis ask yourself:

- Am I clear what the software can do? For example, some CAQDAS claim 'theory building capacities'. But it is the researcher who decides what codes are devised, what functions are operated and what relationships or patterns are significant. For

SPSS users, while the programme will work with the data inputted, it is the role of the researcher to ensure the data has been inputted into the program correctly.

- What is useful about the program in the context of your research project and approach? For example, will you use software as a means of storing, indexing or manipulating data? Or all three?
- What information can I get about the epistemological and explanatory logic of the software from the published information, demonstration guides and formal/informal electronic networks?
- Does the software suit my IT, time and training resources?
- What are my reasons for not using CAQDAS? Am I being technology phobic?

Analytical strategies

Coding your data

Coding involves labelling and categorising your data. For qualitative data, codes represent ways of categorising chunks of data and offer a shorthand label for larger sections of data. For quantitative data, codes can represent different types of responses to social survey research questions. The codes chosen can be derived from conceptual frameworks relevant to your research question and area, devised 'a priori' at the stage of questionnaire design so that answers to questions already have a code attached to them and the task of data analysis involves numerically investigating the coded results. Codes can also be attached to data after data collection, as a researcher devises a label to categorise open-ended responses to a questionnaire or sections of transcript data. Overall, there are three types of codes:

- **A priori coding:** codes that refer to concepts generated from the wider research and theoretical debates related to your research topic.
- **Open coding:** codes representing your interpretation of respondents' viewpoints.
- **In-vivo coding:** codes generated using terms that are used by respondents themselves.

Sheelah Flatman Watson describes devising the majority of her codes prior to administering her questionnaire, all of which were recorded in a 'codebook'. Her questionnaire design involved using closed questions (where a respondent chooses between different answers already set out) and open-ended survey questions (where a respondent can write out their own answers using their own words). Some of her 'codes', therefore, were developed through open and in-vivo coding:

I drafted a codebook in the survey design phase, with codes emerging from the possible range of answers given to the questions I had devised. In the data analysis phase I then had to re-develop this coding system to incorporate the open-ended survey answers. This required similar considerations but in relation to different sources. For the a priori coding, I referred to issues raised in the literature and practitioner debates. For the open coding I was concerned – Were the codes a fair and reasonable description of the meanings within the data? It was a very time-consuming exercise requiring patient readings of each contribution to decipher appropriate categorisation.

Qualitative approaches often involve developing codes inductively. Here codes represent central aspects of a sentence, phrase or a few sentences within a transcript. Codes can be developed in relation to respondents or observational settings viewed as 'cases' or as themes emerging across cases or transcripts. Strategies towards this process include: generating an initial set of codes, re-working coding towards a coding framework, coding your data and analysing relationships between coded data. Initially, researchers often take a cross section of their transcripts or documents, read through the transcripts and begin to label sections of the data using open, in-vivo or some a priori derived codes. If coding is performed manually on printed out documents, different coloured highlighter pens can be used to denote different codes. However, beyond some fairly simple coding this task may become very cumbersome and CAQDAS have facilities for highlighting and labelling text as 'open or in-vivo codes'. Other concepts derived from your reading may seem pertinent to what is being portrayed in your interviews and these can also become codes. Harriet Churchill offers an example of how she generated some codes related to 'coping' in her research on parenting:

Many interviewees discussed their commitment to coping; their experiences of coping and their difficulties. However, the code of 'coping' is too broad and so I tried to devise codes that demonstrate the different facets of coping. The codes that emerged were: coping strategy, services and coping, social support and coping and good motherhood and coping. Some of these codes were generated from the data but others were derived from conceptual debates in the literature around parenting on a low income. Once the codes were devised and all the data indexed, all the data coded as related to coping could be analysed. Codes were subsequently refined and further questions were asked about coping.

As you read through your data, keep asking yourself: what issue is being discussed here; what perspective or concern is the interviewee presenting? Codes should also be clearly defined (CAQDAS have in-built logs for this purpose), mutually exclusive and can be categorised according to overall theme with sub-themes/categories. After reading a selection of transcripts, you will probably already have a long list of codes and categories. It will be worth examining this list once it gets beyond twenty or so codes and thinking about overlaps and connections between codes. Further subsequent rounds of reading transcripts, applying and modifying codes and thinking through the connections between codes can then be performed in order to generate a coding framework. Once you have developed all your codes and these have been arranged into a coding framework, you can then index all your data using these codes. This organises and categories your data into what Mason has called 'bags of data' which can then be analysed further towards deriving explanations for your research questions (Mason, 2002).

Many contributors found coding their data surprisingly time-consuming, demanding much concentration, 'boring and repetitive' as well as exciting and challenging. One contributor felt they 'paid more attention to some transcripts than others because of the time of day they were coded, their interest in the topics and their mood at the time'. Breaking up periods of indexing with refining codes, or doing other activities such as checking recent journals in your area for new publications or inputting your bibliography may help.

Moving towards overall research findings

Once your data are categorised into codes, analysis moves towards focusing on explaining these themes and deciphering patterns and relationships between them in ways that return to providing some answers to your research questions. A line of argument is hence developed, as you offer an overall interpretation of your data. Many of our contributors refer to some helpful activities that aided the construction of an argument.

Framework analysis, or other qualitative thematic approaches, often utilise tables, diagrams, charts or matrices to facilitate examining cases or themes. Some contributors also found writing up their data analysis in the form of thematic papers helped them to think through their overall research questions, theoretical frameworks and the patterns emerging in their data. Both of these strategies helped students to investigate overall patterns in their data. Sheelah Flatman Watson also found that writing a paper on her quantitative data analysis helped her to arrive at some overall findings:

Writing a paper was a wonderful way to focus the data. I developed a series of descriptive statistics that wove a path across phase one, the service provider survey data, and followed these findings with comparative findings from phase two, the

(Continued)

service client survey data. The paper had to be submitted by a particular date and the pressure was on to decide on the salient points to be addressed that would give a coherent picture of the data. The paper got written and my data were no longer data but research findings. I now felt I had an idea how I would approach the remainder of the data.

The process of developing an argument is often conveyed as an iterative process of moving between interpretation, data and theoretical explanations. This involves a continual search for evidence and counter-evidence when devising explanations. Critically assessing your developing interpretations against your data evidence and thinking about alternative explanations is a crucial aspect of this process.

Thinking about the claims you can make: issues of validity and reliability

When arriving at your overall research findings you will be engaging with complex issues of validity and reliability. A major debate in qualitative research fields has been recognition of the interpretative nature of research, and the need to provide evidence of how you arrived at your conclusions from the data you generated via a transparent account of your research design, data collection and analysis and interpretation logics, including perhaps a reflexive account of the role of the researcher in the interpretative process. Making claims in quantitative research also involves interpretation. Quantitative research can attempt to extrapolate patterns from representative samples of wider populations. Emily Tanner, however, felt limited in the generalisation claims she could make from her research approach, although by the end of her study she was also aware of the significant contribution her findings could make to her research area:

I've learned that it is very difficult to design a quantitative study based on new data that uses random probability sampling methods and has a sample size large enough to yield high quality reliable data. I did generate results, but since my sample was based on convenience methods, I could not extrapolate my sample estimates to the wider population. Also I could not make reliable arguments about causation, only relationships of association. To identify cause and effect requires a multiple stage design, which is often unfeasible within the funding and time constraints of a doctoral thesis.

You will need to ask yourself about the possibilities of your research approach and analysis for the types of claims you can make, issues on which the suggested reading below offers further deliberation.

▶ You will need to think about your analysis approach during the research design phase and ensure a logical 'fit' between your research questions, approach, data type and claims.

▶ Preparation for data analysis involves labelling, sorting, archiving, transcribing, anonymising data and inputting data into software programs.

▶ Consider using software packages.

▶ Allow plenty of time for data analysis.

▶ Find out about your ethical and data protection responsibilities.

▶ Data analysis can involve coding, indexing and generating explanations.

▶ Devising charts, tables and matrices may enhance your overview of your data and the relationships between codes.

▶ Writing thematic papers may help develop your argument.

▶ Think about what type of claims your research design and approach allow for.

SUGGESTED READING

Cameron, D. (2001) *Working with Spoken Discourse*. London: Sage.

Field, A. (2005) *Discovering Statistics Using SPSS*. London: Sage.

Fielding, J. and Gilbert, N. (2006) *Understanding Social Statistics*. London: Sage.

Fielding, N.G. and Lee, R.M. (1998) *Computer Analysis and Qualitative Research*. London: Sage.

Mason, J. (2002) *Qualitative Researching*, 2nd edn. London: Sage.

Part II
Writing, Publishing and Networking

This second section of the book deals directly with the importance of writing, publishing and networking, which are three core elements of the PhD success. Much of your energies will be spent fathoming out and extending your skills in these areas. Chapter 6 examines writing as both a process and a product that can be started as early as possible. Asking you questions about your own writing style and hang-ups, this chapter provides strategies for managing the writing process, developing an argument and using different styles of writing. Not shying away from acknowledging that many people find writing difficult, we discuss 'writer's block' and think about strategies for moving forward. Chapter 7 is closely linked to the writing process as it highlights the relevance of writing for publication whilst doing a PhD and the steps to take to get a paper published. There are many benefits to timetabling publishing into your work schedule and getting familiar with the peer review process. Much of this can mean learning to deal with criticisms effectively and not taking the comments from reviewers too personally.

Becoming part of the academic culture and circles will mean that networking, whether you love or loathe it, will become an important task. Chapter 8 looks at how and why networking with both peers at your institution as well as others on a regional, national or international scale will be important for your own progress. Thinking about your place in the research community, we highlight how our contributors often found networking an anxious or time-consuming activity that needed effort. We offer suggestions regarding opportunities and networking structures that are easy to enter and show you how these can be fruitful and often an entertaining part of the job.

We wanted to highlight that doing a PhD is not easy and that deadlines infiltrate the process and can often be a source of anxiety, stress and produce feelings of failure. In Chapter 9 we explain how deadlines are part of the timetabling which will keep you on track and get you completed within the set time. Yet here our contributors highlight what can go wrong with deadlines and how months can slip away and the overall project can simply become unmanageable. We discuss realistic time management strategies as well as offer some solidarity from those who have missed the deadline, hopefully to show that things can turn around. The concluding chapter of this section looks towards the end of the PhD process by examining the viva and what happens beyond the PhD. This chapter offers a realistic look at the examination process, often shrouded in mystery and scary legends about the wrath of the examiners, and highlights that the viva is only the beginning of the end. We offer some tips on preparing both long and short term as well as immediately prior to the viva. Thinking about the afterwards stage we take contributors' experiences to examine what needs to be done about getting a job before the viva arrives. Here we offer some useful tips about career planning for those thinking about working in academia or other sectors unrelated to academia.

Chapter 6
Writing Up and Writer's Block

Writing as activity, process and product

Writing can play a central role in your PhD research in four key ways:

- As an activity that aids the formulation of your ideas and expresses them in written form.
- As a part of the creative and analytical thinking process.
- As the central activity that occurs during the production of your final product – the PhD thesis.
- As a major form of assessment.

Thinking about writing in these four ways – as an activity, analytical process, product and form of assessment – encourages the research student to consider a range of issues. First, as an expressive activity, writing involves the act of conveying ideas, descriptions and explanations in the written word form using appropriate grammatical conventions. The activity of writing gets us thinking about what writing consists of and our own perceptions of our writing style, skills, strengths and weaknesses, as well as the similarities and differences between the written word and alternative forms of expressive activities and language use. PhD students will commence their studies with a wide range of experiences and linguistic backgrounds. As an activity, writing becomes a form of linguistic expression to be practised, personalised and mastered over time.

As an expressive activity, writing is also an aid for creative and analytical thinking. Murray (2002) and Wellington et al. (2005) draw on the work of Elbow (1973) who produced a critique of the traditional view of the PhD process as ending with a period of 'writing up'. This phrase suggests that students 'write up' their research as the final stage of undertaking research and after they have formulated their argument. While this approach may work for some PhD students, for others such a view may actually lead to delaying writing until you 'know what you have to say' and being harshly critical of early attempts at 'writing up'. Elbow wonders if students would ever start writing or move past a first draft if they expected merely to 'write their argument/thesis up'. Rather, we can view writing as more of an ongoing process – as a process integral to generating your ideas and arguments.

For PhD research, writing is also about producing a very tangible product – your thesis – which forms a major part of the assessment process. In order to produce your thesis, you will spend much time doing the activity of writing and using writing as part of progressing your ideas towards the final thesis. You will need to be clear about what is required in writing a thesis and the assessment criteria. However, if you find writing, as an activity, process or product, challenging – you are not alone. There is ample evidence that many PhD students, as well as more established academics, often find themselves suffering from a shaky confidence in their writing (see Back, 2004; Murray, 2004; Wellington et al., 2005).

It is never too early to start writing

Several contributors described having difficulties getting started with writing up. Many underlying issues seemed to influence these experiences such as feeling unprepared, too pressed for time or not confident enough to get started:

> I think I put off writing until the third year of my PhD. Although I read a lot, noted down ideas and arguments in the literature and wrote conference papers on specific aspects of my research – I did not pull this all together into an over-arching written piece early enough. I assumed I would put it all together later on in my final 'writing up year'. Looking back I didn't push myself to move towards some overall argument by writing out how my literature, design, data analysis and developing findings fitted together. In the last year, writing up felt so difficult, I felt I had a lot to say but couldn't put it across in a clear way for quite some time. I think a lot of those difficulties were from not doing enough writing earlier on.
> [Harriet Churchill]

With hindsight, Harriet feels she didn't do enough 'argumentative' writing in the first two years of her thesis. Harriet also felt unconfident about writing, uncertain if she had a clear idea of what she wanted to portray and anxious about whether she had analysed her data enough to start writing up. All of these concerns in effect led to delays in writing. Rather, Murray recommends that writing down your ideas should occur from the outset of your research. There are many ways you can utilise different ways of writing as a means of developing ideas and confidence.

BOX 6.1   Early on you could write about:

- What you are interested in and what led you to these research interests.
- Your initial ideas, reading and personal experiences in relation to your research area.
- Your research questions and what you think you might find out.
- Your methodological approach.

Martin Smith discusses the importance of writing as early as possible:

> Once you start your PhD, start writing straight away and continue to write. Even if you're not satisfied with what you've written and know you'll have to change it later, you will feel more confident in your ability to write, and also feel a sense of accomplishment. It will also help to prevent writer's block, which is often caused by keeping too many ideas in the head and not getting each one down on paper.

John Roberts describes his early writing as consisting of research methods essays and projects:

> Much of what I originally wrote in early pieces of coursework from the first year of my PhD ended up in my methodology chapter. On reflection this taught me a valuable lesson – much of what you write throughout your PhD will be of use somewhere further down the line even if initially it does not look to be the case or even if it does not end up in your final PhD draft. These pieces of writing can be used later on in conference papers, articles and book chapters. The rule to adhere to here is never throw away anything you write.

Managing the writing process

During your PhD research you have the opportunity to develop as a regular, skilled and productive writer. The independent and analytical nature of undertaking a PhD will require developing an aptitude for persistence in progressing and focusing your analysis via writing. Common suggestions for taking a proactive approach towards your writing development are listed in Box 6.2.

BOX 6.2   Managing the writing-up process

- Boice (1994) suggests writing at the same time each day or on the same day each week to get into the habit of regular writing.
- Don't wait until you have a block of time to start writing a paper or a chapter – it may never arrive!
- Devise a timetable for writing. Mark out important short-term and long-term milestones, i.e. research proposal deadline, first year progress report and so on. Set yourself weekly and daily goals that fit in with these longer-term objectives.
- Monitor and time your writing production over an hour/day/week or month. Get to know what your writing output is and your writing speed. This information and awareness will help you to make your targets specific, measurable, achievable, realistic and time-scaled (SMART) (Murray, 2002: 21).
- Define a clear purpose to your writing task, i.e. 'I will write for 2 hours every week day or I will define my research topic in 1,000 words'.
- Discuss writing explicitly with your supervisor and gain feedback on the content, style and grammatical standard (peers can also provide useful feedback).
- Think about your writing habits and approach. Are there any areas in which you can gain further training or support?
- Find out about any writing resources, courses or Web-based support for grammar, punctuation, academic writing or writing for other purposes.
- Find out if your university offers a bibliography software package such as Endnote.

Writing as an aid to argument development

This section considers some suggestions for writing as a way of generating ideas and stimulating your thinking. Suggestions from our contributors included the use of prompts, planning and writing thematic papers. For example, Harriet Churchill describes how she would begin a writing session by gathering her thoughts together:

I would start a writing session in several ways. First, I might re-read something I had written previously and then continue to follow up the ideas. Secondly, I would list out some thoughts and then organise them into some sort of plan or structure for writing. Other times I would just free-write for a while.

To get you started in writing up your methodology or working on an aspect of your data analysis, you could prompt yourself with questions or provocative statements. The aim of writing from prompts is to produce short, focused pieces of writing in your own words as a means of accessing your understanding and viewpoints in preparation for longer pieces of writing. Such an approach can also help with writing up your analysis of a journal article, book or body of literature.

Free-writing and generative writing

These approaches to writing can be helpful in getting you started with writing a new chapter or in moving from thematic analysis towards building an argument. The key idea is to write without stopping or editing for a short length of time as a means of getting some ideas down, akin to 'brainstorming'. Free-writing involves writing for five or ten minutes without a prescribed structure (Murray, 2002). You write non-stop in sentences on whatever you want to write about and even moving between several topics if that occurs. Generally this provides a 'freedom' to express yourself without any judgement about the quality of your writing. This is not writing for an external audience, hence the term 'free-writing'. The uses of free-writing can be to warm you up for writing, to identify key themes and topics, to develop a writing habit, to clarify your thoughts, to express your personal thoughts and understandings, to free your writing from immediate editing and to pull thoughts together at any point in the writing process. The exercise will not produce those carefully structured chapters necessary for your final thesis but may get some of your ideas on paper and help you to see what you think about the issues. Generative writing is similar to free-writing in that you write non-stop in sentences for a specific period of time, but you focus on a particular topic and allow others to comment on it. So the key idea is not to edit your work until you have written out a full page or paragraph on a particular issue or topic.

Presenting and describing quantitative data

Writing up PhD research not only entails words but also numbers and numerical data. If you have collected data that is of a quantifiable nature then learning how to describe and present information using quantitative methods will be something you are likely to receive specific training on. This section will just briefly re-cap on some of the basics regarding presenting numerical data.

- The general rule of thumb is that the most suitable method of displaying data sets is by using the simplest graphical presentation.
- With large data sets the first job is to summarise or put it into a meaningful order.
- Deciding on how to present data pictorially through different charts and tables is an important decision that can assist or detract from understanding your argument.
- Dot plots are best for small numbers where there is no frequency.
- Bar and pie charts represent nominal and ordinal data.
- Bar and line charts represent ratio and interval data.
- Histograms represent ratio or interval data that is discrete data with a frequency.
- A cumulative frequency graph is useful for open class intervals.
- Time series graphs can measure an attribute over time.

(adapted from Curnock (1996) *Quantitative Methods in Business*. Cheltenham: Stanley Thornes)

Writing thematic working papers

John Roberts found it useful to write thematic working papers as a means of developing an interpretation of his data:

> I faced the problem of integrating my primary data with my theoretical literature. To be honest, I found this to be the biggest obstacle in finishing my PhD because I had so much data. At this point I felt that the most useful exercise for me to undertake would be to write up as much of the historical material as I could. By focusing on writing up just one section of my data – I was able slowly to piece together the emergence of Speaker's Corner in Hyde Park, London – the object of enquiry of my PhD.

Focusing on writing about one particular set of issues, type of data or thematic consideration may help you to focus your thesis, gain valuable feedback and even begin to draft an article suitable for publication (see Chapter 7).

Writing up your thesis

It is worth finding out about the regulations and conventions associated with a social science doctoral thesis as early as possible. At the beginning of the research writing up your thesis may seem like a long way off, but getting an impression of what is expected and what a thesis looks like and reads like may help to gain a realistic impression.

- Read the doctorate submission regulations produced by your host university. Check details of word length, assessment criteria, assessment procedure and essential content, i.e. What should be on the title page? What chapters are stipulated?
- Ask your supervisor and any other senior academics to suggest examples of a 'good' thesis for you to look at. Ask for their opinion of why the thesis was 'good'. All theses submitted are also available via your university library/thesis database.
- Review the National Committee for Postgraduates and Quality Assurance Agency documents on good practice and thesis assessment.
- Ask any peers that have recently submitted about the assessment process and their experiences of producing their thesis.

Producing the thesis: working on aspects of global planning

A thesis can be viewed as a 'defended integrated argument' that builds on theoretical or empirical work in a particular research area. The argument makes a claim that is placed in the context of other possible counter-claims and ongoing claims by other researchers and authors in the field. In developing your thesis, writing while thinking about 'global planning' will be important. Global planning refers to the bigger picture – your overall questions, argument, audience, purpose and structure. In writing up your thesis, you will need to think about these global aspects and seek a coherent and appropriate thesis for your task and audience. Important questions to ask are:

- What previous work has been done in this area? What are the key arguments and focus of inquiry?
- How does your work relate to this previous work? What do you intend to contribute?
- What is your research question? How similar and different are your central questions to previous work?
- What have you done in your research? What were the stages of your research? Why did you do what you did? And why in that order?
- How did you go about answering your questions?
- What methods and approaches did you use?
- What have you found out? How do your findings add to the previous work?
- What do your findings mean? Do they raise any new questions or refine existing concepts? What further research do you propose?
- Who is my audience? What do I know about them? How should I write appropriately for the audience?

Sheelah Flatman Watson found writing conference papers helped her to be disciplined in her writing with tight deadlines to meet. Planning such a step-by-step approach towards a final thesis may help in establishing and getting past important milestones on the way through writing up your thesis:

> Writing a conference paper meant that the pressure was on to decide on the salient points to be addressed that would serve the respondent community well and give a coherent picture of the research. My supervisor reviewed and critiqued the paper. After this presentation, I was then invited to prepare a plenary paper for a forthcoming international conference, three weeks away. Again, engaging the data to produce a follow on paper guided the research further. Having deadlines to meet for the paper made decision-making purposeful within a limited timeframe. Questions from the audience helped me refine my arguments.

Working on the specifics of each chapter

As well as thinking about the 'global' picture, you will need to think about the specific contribution each paragraph, page and chapter makes to the overall thesis. In writing your chapters you can use generative writing and free-writing to get some ideas out. Also you may want to plan out your ideas in a diagram or in a list. Try not to edit too excessively at the beginning – try to get at least a page or two down first.

> I would often start a session of writing by editing the paragraphs and pages I had already written. In hindsight I realised I could spend half a day doing this as I preciously thought through each sentence trying to get it totally right. I then tended to run up against a deadline before I had completed a first draft of a chapter or paper. The problem then was that I had little time left for re-drafting and I found it hard to let go of paragraphs I had spent so long working on.
> [Harriet Churchill]

Think about the flow of a chapter. Most chapters require an overall introduction letting the reader know what issues and areas will be covered. Use sub-headings to indicate how the overall area will be discussed via a number of more specific discussions. Signpost the reader along the way with reminders of what you have covered so far, where you are heading and what relationship your specific point has to the overall chapter and thesis. Allow plenty of time for editing. During the editing process think about the 'flow' of your ideas, grammatical accuracy and the clarity of expression.

Writer's block and strategies for moving on

'Writer's block' is a general term used to describe the feeling of being stuck in your writing. Many contributors described having 'bad writing days', feeling 'unable to write' or being very dissatisfied by their 'written work'. Indeed such days appear common among all writers, no matter the level of experience or subject. The bad writing days could be the ones where you sit at your computer, get easily distracted, feel negative about the quality of your writing or spend all day writing one paragraph. John Roberts describes writer's block as emerging from uncertainty about the connections between two aspects of his data:

I had been experiencing some difficulty about how I was going to integrate my ethnographic data with both my theoretical and historical data. In many respects this is where I had encountered what might be thought of as writer's block. I had difficulty in thinking through how all of my ethnographic material could be used in a coherent manner with what I had now written. The solution, however, was a quick and easy one. I realised that I had already written more than enough words for the PhD. I thereby decided not to include the ethnography but to try to return to it after my PhD viva by writing separate papers on it.

BOX 6.3 Overcoming writer's block

- Ask yourself whether you are suffering from writer's block. Is your writing moving forward slowly? Do you feel demoralised or confused? Are you bored? Are you being overly critical when judging your earlier writing?
- Try free-writing or generative writing about your thesis in general or a chapter or issue just to get some writing done.
- Try to express your ideas verbally (record this if possible) or visually in a diagram before sitting down to write.
- Re-read your previous writing.
- Take a break, go for a walk, leave your paper for a few days, work on something such as your bibliography or start on another chapter.
- Break your writing sessions up and schedule some rewards for any small or large achievements, e.g. an afternoon or day off for each chapter completed.
- Develop a regular habit of writing.

▶ Writing forms a central part of your thesis production but can also be an aid to analytical and creative thinking and help develop your expressive skills.

▶ Think about how you see yourself as a writer. How do you feel about academic writing for your doctorate?

▶ Start writing as early as possible and try to develop a regular habit of writing.

▶ Use writing to stimulate ideas through the use of free-writing or generative writing.

▶ Manage the writing process – set yourself long-term and short-term goals.

▶ Seek advice on availability and the use of a bibliographic software package.

▶ Think about writing short thematic papers to aid argument development.

▶ Think about capitalising on your writing – can you turn any thematic papers into journal articles?

▶ Find out about the conventions and expectations for your thesis structure and content.

▶ In writing up your thesis, think about the global picture (argument and message) and the structure/specific contribution of each chapter.

▶ Seek advice and feedback on your writing.

▶ Allow for plenty of time for re-drafting.

SUGGESTED READING

Brause, R.S. (2000) *Writing Your Doctoral Dissertation: Invisible Rules for Success*. London: Falmer.

Dunleavy, P. (2003) *Authoring a PhD Thesis: How to Plan, Draft, Write and Finish a Doctoral Dissertation*. Basingstoke: Palgrave.

Elliot, R. and Lawler, G. (2006) *Your PhD Thesis: How to Plan, Draft, Revise and Edit Your Thesis*. London: Studymates.

Murray, R. (2002) *How to Write a Thesis*. Maidenhead: Open University Press.

Thody, A. (2006) *Writing and Presenting Research*. London: Sage.

Chapter 7

Papers and Publishing

▶ The place of publishing in the lifecourse of the doctorate
▶ The options of where to publish and how to decide the best readership
▶ The benefits of getting your work published early
▶ A brief overview of the publication process for journals
▶ How to deal with challenging remarks and turn criticism into a successful publication
▶ The link between publishing, networking and presenting at conferences

Why the rush?

Increasingly, writing for publication as part of the PhD process is becoming a necessity as the competition for academic jobs tightens and the weight given to peer reviewed publications remains significant since the introduction of the Research Assessment Exercise. Whatever form academic assessment takes in the future, those interested in a research or academic career must take publishing seriously from an early stage. In addition, an integral part of working towards a doctorate is presenting your work to others, whether this be peers in postgraduate workshops, your mentor in supervision sessions, or an internal panel at various 'upgrade' stages. Publishing a piece of written work is the final stage of this process of presenting your findings, arguments, theories and methodological reflections to the wider academic community. As Becker (2004: 143) remarks, some of the reasons to go for publication include extending your writing skills, but getting your work published can also be a great motivator.

Traditional academic cultures did not usually encourage students to seek publication. This has changed significantly over the past decade as publication has been the benchmark through which individuals are judged. This chapter explores why you should get involved with publishing before you have been given the golden seal of approval through doctorate success. This can be answered by thinking about content, confidence, criticisms and careers.

Content

In terms of content, hopefully you already have interesting things to say before you submit the thesis and are enthusiastic to report what you have found. Many of the contributors described now they siphoned off specific and discrete research findings from their PhD and prepared them for a journal article both before and after submitting the thesis.

Even if you can get to the stage where you can write a coherent paper, there will still be doubts about entering the publishing world. Jonny Burnett expresses some typical doubts when he describes his thinking about writing for publication in his first year: 'Although ideas were certainly there, they were accompanied by reservations regarding their validity, and whether I had the ability to structure and present them coherently.' You need to be sure that you have something that is worthwhile to say, that it is not a repetition of knowledge already out there and that your information is accurate and thorough. For example, the basic tenets of the piece must contribute to moving a debate forward, reporting new findings, addressing current policy issues or dealing with a contemporary event. Assessing whether your paper contributes to knowledge is a matter for your own judgement and asking your supervisors. As we will discuss, the peer reviewers will also have plenty to say about originality.

Confidence

Dipping your toe in the world of peer review is a daunting experience and one of the main barriers is normally confidence. Doug Morrisson reflects on this: 'The time to start thinking about publishing is highly individualistic … . I was initially put off by lack of confidence, fear of criticism and concerns about originality.' You can only gain confidence by going through the process, so don't let this be the reason for delay. One way to build confidence is by doing your homework in terms of checking out potential journals. Becker (2004: 145) summarises: 'Each journal has its own bias in terms of the type of article in which it is interested. This might be historical bias, an editorial angle, or a preference for highly theoretical articles.' It is important to think where your work would fit in. For example, some journals are slanted towards quantitative work, while others have reputations for publishing qualitative material or more theory-based arguments.

Criticism

Believe it or not, you will be well used to receiving critical feedback about your work long before you receive comments back from the peer review process. Part of the PhD journey is about receiving criticism, working with it and developing your ideas. Receiving critical feedback is not just about being a PhD student, but is the process of being an academic and producing empirical findings and theoretical argument that drips into the pot of knowledge. John Roberts found that the publishing process was very helpful whilst writing up the thesis because it enabled connections to be made between the findings and the literature as well as providing guidance on the structure of the PhD:

> While I was writing up I had also written two papers that I submitted to journals as well as a book chapter on ethnographic methods. One of these journal articles along with the book chapter was especially useful in making me think about structuring the PhD. By focusing upon a specific part of the thesis I was forced to look at legal statements in some detail. Indeed, external referee reports had requested that I do so before the article was published. By doing so I was forced to make more explicit links with my theoretical material, particularly around the work of radical and Marxist theories of the state and law and around the work of a group of discourse theorists I drew upon called the Bakhtin Circle. This really was an important turning point in my writing up experience because it helped to bring together different threads of my PhD.

Playing the publishing game is very much about learning to use criticism constructively to reach the desired goal and not slumping into a corner never to submit a piece of work again! Rejection is all part of the process.

BOX 7.1

Learning to deal with peer review is an important skill and will benefit your PhD as well as your career. So don't delay, get publishing today!

Career

The other reason to get on with publishing relates to getting a job. If you want an academic career then it is essential that you timetable writing for publication into your doctorate. If you are not intending to stay within academia then publishing during your doctorate is not as important but more about personal satisfaction rather than career ladders. When applying for an academic post your CV will be scanned for experience of teaching, research and publishing. If you haven't got publishing experience then someone else will have and you may not get the interviews.

Getting your work out there

Timing

There are no set rules for when you publish material from your PhD. It is very exceptional to be able to publish material from your MA degree, and usually doctoral students begin to think about publication in the second or third year. Some people have in mind two or three articles they would like to get out of their thesis either towards the end of writing up or later. Others decide they want to try to turn the thesis into a monograph at the end of the process. Although turning a thesis into a book is becoming increasingly difficult because publishers don't make much money from specialist books, it is possible through smaller publishers and specialist presses. Journals sometimes invite submissions to special issues, so look out for the 'calls for papers'. Also, PhD students may be asked to write chapters for edited collections. This is a useful way to begin the publishing process, as although the chapter will still go through an editorial process, this is an opportunity for supportive feedback and a fairly guaranteed successful outcome.

What and where to publish

Wisker (2001: 316) advises postgraduates to consider carefully why to publish, where to publish and what to publish. Important questions indeed. Deciding *what* you want to publish needs to be done in conjunction with *where* you want to publish. There are many different types of academic and non-academic routes to publication that are common amongst PhD students. Journals are the place for lengthier traditional papers (approximately 8,000 words), but there are also opportunities for 'observations', or 'methodological reflection' and 'review essays' that tend to be shorter. Marta Bolognani found one of the less conventional publishing options was a real boost early on in her PhD:

> If you are keen on circulating some preliminary research findings but you have not contextualised them appropriately in a theoretical framework, you could consider writing 'research notes'. Research notes are based on your empirical findings and have a word length reduced in comparison to articles (usually 3,000 words). This would get your name out in a journal without having to wait to finish writing your thesis, and the review process would normally be significantly shorter than for an article.

Jonny Burnett has successfully used non-academic publishing outlets for his preliminary findings: 'There are a variety of magazines, pamphlets and booklets which are much more suited to shorter and more direct commentaries, which may have a far wider (and more relevant) readership.' These avenues are not to be discounted, but remember there is a hierarchy to types of publications. It is fairly common to write co-authored pieces with others during your PhD; this may be other academics you have networked with or other PhD students. However, be clear from the start what the order of authorship is: you don't want to do all the work and then be relegated to second author. Second author is fine as long as the division of labour reflects this. It is worth taking note of the hierarchy of writing relationships when you are thinking about what to do next and which offers of co-writing will be fruitful.

The basic ranking order in terms of prestige is as follows:

1 Single authored book
2 Single authored journal article in peer reviewed international journal
3 Joint authored journal article in peer reviewed international journal. Here 'joint' refers to an equal amount of input into the writing of the article and usually the whole research project. This normally refers to two authors
4 Co-authored book
5 Edited book
6 Second author of journal article in peer reviewed international journal. Here 'second author' can refer to several authors who have all had some level of input into the research and writing. For instance, you could have been involved in the data analysis and appear on a paper as a second author
7 Chapter in edited book
8 Grey material such as reports or magazines
9 Working papers or conference proceedings

BOX 7.2   Choose where you send your article carefully

Think about the following:

• What is the readership or audience that your paper speaks to?
• Are traditional journals the best place to publish at this stage?
• Could you begin with a more specialist publication or non-academic format?

Although not ranked on the hierarchy of publishing formats, given the often daunting nature of writing and, more so, the peer review process, there are several journals specifically for postgraduates across the country. Most of these journals are not specific to students studying in the host institution but are open to all. The group **Esharp** (electronic social sciences and arts review for postgraduates, www.sharp.arts. gla.ac.uk) provides a list of institutions that host postgraduate journals including:

- **Postgraduate Forum** – e-journal based at the School of Historical Studies, The University of Newcastle www.ncl.ac.uk/historical/postgrad_forum/
- **ManuScript** – English and American studies

Marta Bolognani's first experience of publishing is a useful example of the process, highlighting that a published piece of work has a lengthy history before it is sent for review:

> I presented the first draft of the paper at a workshop and once I worked around the feedback received I sent it off to a journal. The first attempt was a failure, but the anonymous peer reviewers still had to write extensive comments on why they thought the paper was not suitable for publication. Once I implemented the changes they suggested, I was able to send the paper off to another journal. This process can take a long time, especially because you are forbidden from sending your paper off to more than one journal at a time.

Often, final published papers start their life as 'work in progress' and are presented informally to peers (often in departmental seminars) or more formally at conferences. The paper is then 'worked up' into a full article before sending it to the peer review process.

Writing it!

Once you have decided where the article is going, you need to write it. Do this to your best ability, but don't stagnate due to lack of confidence. After a couple of publications in what is known as 'grey literature' (newsletters, websites, magazines, campaign literature), Jonny Burnett noted that a pattern of procrastination can set in if your confidence is suffering a little. He advises: 'If thinking about writing a paper for publication then perhaps the best advice is to simply "get on with it". There is a point where drafting and making notes must give way to the actual writing process.' You need to crack on also because of the amount of time it takes to go through the review process. Initial attempts to write a journal article may take a few months. The review process (from submission to publication) can take anywhere between 6 and 18 months, so consider this timescale in your PhD timetabling. However, as Gina Wisker advises, 'beware that you might be sacrificing the coherence of your thesis to a desire to get in print' (2001: 317). Time management is crucial here and a balance between writing the thesis and writing for publication must be achieved.

It may be that you have something already written. Teela Sanders found her thesis was too long, so she omitted a set of findings, changed the thesis chapter into a journal article (quite a big task which took about a month) and submitted to a journal. Rugg and Petre (2004: 83) pinpoint the literature review as a place to start: 'If you have done the literature review for your PhD properly, then it should be publishable as a review paper.' However, speaking from experience of rejection, make sure you do not simply bung the literature review chapter into a journal. It must be re-formatted as a coherent article and to the style and audience of the journal. This is likely to involve reframing your argument so that the article 'speaks' to the readership and does not sound like a thesis chapter. Write the article in the journal's house style, sticking to word length, referencing format etc. This information is always on the journal's homepage under titles such as 'information for authors', 'notes for contributors', or 'author guidelines'. Make sure you apply these guidelines, as articles can be sent back if they are not in the house style.

BOX 7.3

Be serious from the outset about your writing. You should only submit a piece that is of your highest standard. Do not submit a piece of work before someone you respect has considered it.

The publishing process

The process of reviewing an article in a traditional journal follows this standard procedure:

1   Submit paper to a journal. Nowadays this is usually done electronically but check for specifics.
2   The editor will read the paper and decide if it is within the remit of the journal.
3   If so, it will be sent out to (at least) two anonymous reviewers normally related to your field. This is called the 'peer review' process and almost all journals use this to determine which articles are suitable, original and publishable.
4   They will return comments to the editor. You will receive a set of comments which are anonymous and normally a summary of changes from the editor. The level of commentary is very arbitrary ranging from a couple of sentences to a review of your paper paragraph by paragraph correcting typos and grammar as well as the argument. Also, the editor will have reviewed these comments and will write to you with the outcome.
5   The options are usually (1) rejection; (2) major corrections, revise and resubmit; (3) resubmit with minor corrections; (4) acceptance. Bearing in mind that most journals reject over 70% of articles submitted, if you get 'revise and resubmit' you are a winner. Make sure you take this opportunity to address the main criticisms and resubmit

within the allocated time. When you resubmit make sure you send a covering letter stating the changes you have made and how you have addressed the feedback.

6   If the paper is rejected, use the criticisms to redraft and submit elsewhere. Don't despair – this is normal and happens to *all* academics.

7   Once you have resubmitted it the paper may either go just to the editor, or it may be sent to review again. This process is usually quicker and you will receive some final comments before publication.

8   When the final version has been confirmed the paper then goes to the copy editor who will check for spelling, grammar and referencing inaccuracies. You will get a checklist of corrections, which normally have to be turned around in days.

9   Finally, the proofs will be sent to you for checking (online) and signing the copyright form.

10   Congratulations, you are a published academic!

BOX 7.4   Do your market research

Study the editorial objectives to make sure your work fits and read a couple of articles in the journal to get an idea of the writing style, structure and type of material presented.

They said what? be prepared for challenging comments

Rugg and Petre (2004: 215) advise 'aim to have about 75 per cent of your papers rejected'. We are slightly more optimistic than this but at the same time you should still be aware that academic publishing is a very tough game. The comments that are returned to you can take the form of helpful, insightful pointers on how to make the paper into a publishable piece that makes maximum impact, or comments can be simply unhelpful. Marta Bolognani explains:

Some of the comments can be very harsh and not expressed with consideration of the feelings of the authors, but the pain can really be worth it if the critique is constructive … . Anonymous peer review from a journal, whether they accept your article for publication or not, offers the opportunity to receive comments from people who are 'experts' in your field.

Always look through the comments for the positive. Jonny Burnett's experience sums up how to deal with an article that is rejected:

> Almost all authors have at some point had work turned down for publication. If (when) this happens it is worth taking time to think clearly why this was the case. Perhaps the paper simply was not of publishable standard, and if this is so then it may be necessary to redraft and think about what aspects of the paper were of use and could be incorporated elsewhere. However, it is also useful to consider whether the publication itself was the 'right place' to have the work presented.

BOX 7.5

It is very hard not to, but don't take harsh comments personally. Sift out the useful feedback from the comments that say more about the reviewer than your paper.

As previously indicated, there is a significant chance that you will be asked to 'revise and resubmit' the article to the same journal. In this scenario, the editor will have considered the reviewers' comments and summarised the most important changes that need to be made before publication. However, this is great news because it usually signifies that the article will be published subject to making the changes. Doug Morrison offers his experience of this:

> I had been invited to resubmit subject to re-formatting and some corrections. Moreover, the reviewers had made numerous comments that ranged from structural and referencing advice to material that I had not considered and which they felt my work would potentially benefit from.

Taken in the right spirit, reviewers' comments can be one of the few opportunities for direct commentary on your work.

Remember that once an article bearing your name has been published your work may reach a range of different readerships and you are potentially opening the floodgates to criticism from the wider community. Jonny Burnett reflects on responses he and his co-authors received from academics and other readers after their work had 'gone public':

> After one short article was made available on the Internet the responses were varied and diverse. Some took the form of personal insults, others warm praise. Either way, hearing responses to written work is a useful experience and helps the author to reflect on what was said – even if this still results in wholehearted disagreement.

Once your work is given the seal of 'peer review' approval you are considered a serious player in your field and this will attract attention and hopefully discussion and networking. Doug Morrison found his publication sparked interest from others respected in the field:

> Since publication I have benefited from a variety of correspondence, some very positive, supporting my work and some of course disagreeing vehemently. The important thing is that responses from others generated discussion, some of which has provided me with new insights into my area of research and caused me to pause for thought and to reconsider some perspectives again.

Like supervision sessions, comments from reviewers can be useful and others are hardly worth reading as they muddle, confuse and sometimes upset. Don't let any of these revelations put you off. We all have to go through it and the sooner you get started the quicker you can learn to manage this part of the academic process.

Linking networking, conferences and publishing

Finally, it is important to think about publishing alongside engaging with conferences and other forms of networking. We have dedicated the next chapter specifically to this part of the doctoral experience, because if you want to become part of the academic community you need to network. Writing a paper for publication (in whatever format) should be strategically linked to presenting a paper at a conference and networking with like-minded researchers, writers, policymakers and practitioners. Publishing before your doctorate is completed is a significant time management task and the whole endeavour should not detract from the priority of getting those chapters written. That is why thinking strategically about what to present at a conference should be done with publications in mind. Marta Bolognani's advice is a useful guide to how these tasks are interlinked:

Start from a presentation at a conference, then use the feedback received from the audience to make changes to the paper and then send the paper to a journal. The whole process can be enlightening and help develop your thoughts.

By presenting your findings or ideas at conferences and workshops your name gets known by the relevant academic circles and it is then that you start making links with kindred spirits. Becoming part of a network (even if this ends up being a chat in the pub, or on an email list), enables you to ask someone in your area to have a look at an article before you publish, or even start on a joint venture together. Feedback from conferences about your work is helpful when writing a paper. Doug Morrison notes how feedback from conferences and being part of a network can help with broader thinking processes:

Such correspondence has provided me with the opportunity to network with colleagues from a variety of different backgrounds who also share a similar area interest. Such cross-fertilisation has proved to be a very positive experience and has helped with my PhD.

Remember that giving a conference paper is also about taking questions and entering into a discussion – this is useful feedback to work into your paper. Of course, once you have a publication, whether it be in *The Big Issue*, a NGO website or a top-ranked journal, getting your name out there enhances your networking opportunities.

BOX 7.6

Completing your PhD should be the main priority, but if you are keen to disseminate your work, you could take a month out to write a piece for a journal. Seek your supervisor's advice.

Key Points to Remember

▶ If you are thinking of an academic career then publishing during your PhD should be a timetabled activity.
▶ Be strategic about what conferences you attend and the papers you present. Try to work up a conference presentation into an article.

- ▶ When choosing *where* to send your work do your homework on the journal.
- ▶ Get someone you trust to read the article before you submit – not your mum who will love it whatever you write! This could be your supervisor, another academic in your field. But again, don't show them a sloppy unfinished version – their time is precious too.
- ▶ Only submit a paper that you think is 'at it's best'. Sloppiness annoys editors.
- ▶ Expect to make revisions. No one gets a paper accepted without making some changes, and with this comes sometimes harsh comments.
- ▶ Don't give up. If the paper is rejected – learn from the comments and submit elsewhere. If you are asked to 'revise and resubmit' you are halfway to victory. Do what the editors ask within the time limit – and taste the success.
- ▶ Remember you are new to all of this – it takes time to learn the publishing game. But what does practice make …?

SUGGESTED READING AND RESOURCES

Boice, R. (1994) *How Writers Journey to Comfort and Fluency: A Psychological Adventure.* London: Praeger.

Murray, R. (2004) *Writing for Academic Journals.* Maidenhead: Open University Press.

Rugg, G. and Petre, M. (2004) *The Unwritten Rules of PhD Research.* Maidenhead: Open University Press. Chapter 8 'Writing'.

Esharp (electronic social sciences and arts review for postgraduates) www.sharp.arts.gla.ac.uk

Chapter 8
Networking

It's good to talk: the value of networking

Networking consists of 'initiating and maintaining social relationships for professional related purposes' and can involve face–to–face, postal or internet based communication (Arnold, 1997: 83). While some people seem adept at networking, others shudder at what can appear very instrumental motivations for getting to know other people. For Jonny Burnett networking has 'connotations of careerism' where interactions are about 'insincere backslapping, laughing falsely at poor jokes or angling for new opportunities'. However, networking, when based on mutual respect and reciprocity, can enhance your professional life, working environment and research activities as you gain new insights and share experiences, ideas and knowledge. Whatever you feel about networking, whatever your experiences to date and whether you think you are any good at it – there is no detracting from the potential value networking in progressing and enhancing your research ideas and career. Benefits can be:

- Gaining practice in verbally presenting, articulating and defending your ideas.
- Finding out about new areas of inquiry or being presented with intellectual challenges.
- Finding out about what other research and activities are being conducted in your area.
- Finding out about job or further research opportunities.
- Meeting 'gatekeepers' or other significant people who can enable you to continue with your research or put you in touch with research participants.

- Meeting others who may become professional colleagues or even friends.
- Feeling part of a wider community that shares a particular research or campaigning purpose.
- Feeling valued and active as part of a wider community.

Sheelah Flatman Watson felt her networking activities were instrumental to her intellectual development and also found engaging in networks across several disciplines helped her to gain a wider perspective of her research topic:

> Networking across the academic disciplinary and practitioner communities, I believe, was key to my understanding of a variety of perspectives – contextualising parental and practitioner perspectives and the phenomenon being researched. Attending a variety of gatherings and getting in touch with different groups and individuals, gave me a broader understanding of the issues being addressed at the various levels of the community.

Anxious about networking?

Although many appreciate the potential value of networking, many doctoral students can still feel uncomfortable or uncertain about how to proceed. It is extremely common for postgraduates to feel anxious about networking in the context of getting to know a research community and feeling a 'junior' member. For example, in the first year of her PhD study, Marta Bolognani vividly remembers attending her first national conference where 'some of the most famous names in her discipline were present'. Attending such an event and coming face to face with senior academics whom she had admired and whose work she respected produced a mixture of emotions and aspirations. While Marta wanted to 'meet the people who had written such crucial books for my academic development', she also felt 'uncertain and daunted' at the thought of approaching them:

> I did not want to seem a 'groupie'. I did not want to be seen to be 'blowing my own trumpet' either. I also did not have anything, I assumed, that would have been of interest to them to 'exchange' for conversation. In practice, though, I was quite surprised about the welcoming attitudes of most of the academics. I learnt that they are keen on networking too.

Where is my research community?

You may wonder if there is a research community that fits your research interests and how to access such a community. In the early days of networking you may feel like the outsider, with uncertainty about these issues, your worth and place in a larger research community. Taking a proactive and reciprocal approach will help overcome these concerns. Don't wait for others to identify themselves or confirm your value and inclusion – you are unlikely to receive any personal invitations to a well-defined research community! Shelaah Flatman Watson remembers feeling the 'outsider' and without a 'research community' for quite some time due to several reasons:

> In the early days of my PhD, as a mature student, I have often felt out of step with fellow attendees in various forums. I am not the typical research student. But also, at the service based practitioner gatherings I was not a service provider. Neither was I a service user, nor the parent of a service user. Where do I fit in? I have felt people were suspicious of my position. I have learned that there is a distrust of researchers and a cynicism towards any forms of bureaucracy, management or outsiders.

This prompted Shelaah to think through her role and research community quite carefully. She offers valuable advice on 'the importance of thinking through how you present yourself in such contexts and what you can bring to interactions'. She found 'listening, engaging in ways that are sensitive to the political and social context, and taking a genuinely interested and empathetic approach' helped her to connect with 'the most reluctant service providers who could change their view of me to friend rather than foe, and respect the research work that I was embarking on even though I was documenting the experiences of the clients they serve'.

BOX 8.2 Thinking about research communities and your relationship to them

Ask yourself:

- Are there any collective professional groups within your research area?
- Would you be able to contribute to or learn from these groups? In what ways?
- Do you feel an outsider in particular collective professional settings? Why may this be the case? What would be an appropriate way of getting involved?
- How can you introduce yourself to a wider community? How can you present your research interests and motivations?
- Are there additional (non-academic) ways you are willing and able to contribute? Can you get involved in some voluntary or administration work for example?

Networking is about giving as much as receiving

Building trusting and reciprocal networking relationships takes time and effort. An apparently hostile response can have a valid non–personal explanation and help you to think about the history to the relationships established across your research community. Being aware of this history and context can help you to think about your approach and activities in a more informed way. Sheelah Flatman Watson's example also illustrates how networking can be based on mutually reciprocal exchange – summed up by the phrase 'give and take'. This involves considering what contribution you can make and what motivates your getting involved. The beauty of networking is the resources each person brings to any exchange, whether these be attentiveness, interest, a list of contacts, information or ideas – and how the sharing of such resources has multiple benefits. Marta Bolognani took this strategy on wholeheartedly in her aspirations to be as useful to others as they had been to her:

When you come back from conferences tidy up your notes so you have the contact details and the research interests of an academic. If you do not need them then someone else might. I can remember meeting two people working on the same research area at two different conferences, I passed on their details to each other and they established an exchange of ideas! When you pass on somebody else's contact, though, make sure that it is OK with both parties.

Jonny Burnett, on the other hand, felt his role as an academic networking across policy, political, academic and practitioner communities enabled him to contribute to 'breaking down barriers between academic and non-academic networks' generating forms of shared understanding and 'forging links between different organisations, bodies and activities'. Within the generation of reciprocal professional relationships you will also need to be selective to some extent. Not only are there some who do not share in the vision or practices of reciprocity – you will need to make sure you can deliver and are committed to any offers of help and support you provide – equally you need to be able to decline offers and opportunities when the completion of your thesis must take priority!

Taking a proactive approach

Taking a proactive approach to networking involves taking time to plan, prepare and find out about networking opportunities. The following sections discuss opportunities and avenues to pursue.

Peer networking

Networking with other postgraduate and research students may be a good place to start. As Marta Bolognani noted, you can start from 'thinking small' as 'sometimes other PhD students can be even more important to your work than the most senior academic in your field' as they are also immersed in recent debates. You may be familiar with the research being undertaken by your fellow peers within your research unit, but have you explored similar areas of interest across departmental or disciplines areas? You may not want to 'talk work' with your peers all the time but are you aware of their research interests and activities? Who do they network with? What research issues are they dealing with? What networking events do they attend and what is their experience of them?

Networking within your university

Your own university can provide numerous networking opportunities. A fairly obvious starting place would be within your supervisory team or departmental corridors. Getting to know and attending events happening within your department may well already be part of your normal working routine. These events can be valuable for finding out about individual and collective research interests, priorities and activities. Several universities hold regular postgraduate and departmental seminars. Beyond this, as Jonny Burnett soon realised, 'academics tend to know many other academics and are frequently pleased to both introduce others to colleagues and friends who have knowledge in particular areas, and to inform people of relevant research'. It may be an idea to:

- Find out about the members of your department and university – what are members' research interests and activities?
- Ask your supervisor about the conferences, events and associational groups they attend.
- Show your interest in networking with other academics in your field.
- Suggest hosting a small event together or within your department.
- Seek out researchers elsewhere in the university who are engaged in similar research.

JK Tina Basi reminds us of the enhancement to our social lives in general through active involvement in the activities of the host university:

> Remember that networking is not just about work. Networking is also about adding a social dimension to your academic life. Do your best to attend gatherings or events in your department and at your university. Meeting people in a social setting can often establish friendly relationships that will help to dilute the isolation or loneliness you may feel during the course of your PhD. And don't forget about virtual networking! There are many opportunities on the Internet to learn of people's work and most provide relevant contact details should you want to get in touch.

Sheelah Flatman Watson had the opportunity to take part in social events that were organised by her university such as the research students' 'weekend away'. This weekend was organised for all first year students, involved students from many universities and was structured around 'presenting your research proposal and building a research student community'. If you find there are no organised postgraduate events in your university can you suggest or help establish one?

Seminars, conferences and research networks

Seminars, conferences and research workshops or ongoing networks are the most prominent forms of networking among academic communities. Marta Bolognani approached her academic field as a set of individuals, organisations and communities as well as an area of academic knowledge and arguments. This involved actively:

> Going through and reviewing the literature I was reading and then noting on an on-going basis who the contemporary researchers in the field were, both at home and abroad. I joined organisations active in the community including service provider organisations, client group organisations and groups of academics collaborating under varied umbrella organisations.

When reading literature or researching an issue make a note of where researchers are based and key associations and organisations operating in your research area. Jonny Burnett then proceeded by approaching academics directly:

> I have benefited from simply contacting people working in a field that I am researching and asking if they have time to discuss their research. Although this is perhaps rather a blunt approach, I have found that many people are prepared to do this even when busy with other commitments.

Attending and presenting papers at conferences and seminars provides a major arena for networking. If you haven't already done so, you can find out about the funding opportunities within your department for research students to attend seminars and conferences. Several conferences offer subsidised registration fees for students and travel expenses so check out the funding opportunities before you decide it is too costly. Your supervisor may have valuable advice as to the most prominent and smaller scale conferences and seminars to attend in your area. Take the plunge – present a paper – this will enable you to discuss your work with other academics.

You may prefer smaller conferences, workshops or discussion groups/networks to larger conferences. The first issue will be to find out what forms these take in your research area. Searches on the Web, asking your supervisor and asking other academics may be fruitful lines of inquiry. Marta Bolognani found two research networks relevant to her research area. Marta offered her support to one network through attendance and then taking on some voluntary work within the group:

> I took on some of the administrative tasks that can easily be dealt with by post-graduate students. Tasks such as collecting names and details and then sending them around the participants in the days after the conference can be a good way to network and not to go unnoticed. In this way you do not have to think about a network strategy as you will have the chance to chat with people while you are doing your administrative task. Volunteering is also a good way to avoid paying conference fees and have free meals if you are on a tight budget!

Non-academic groups, discussion lists and events

As we discussed earlier, building bridges between academic and non–academic interest groups can also be an important and valuable form of networking. Networking can provide an endless list of possible people and organisations that can contribute to your understanding of the issues in your area, can gain from your research contributions and expand your social networks of interesting people and personalities! These outcomes were valued by Jonny Burnett, who here describes his engagement with campaigning groups:

In my experience various campaigners and activists are also willing to share ideas and collaborate in projects. Moreover, this frequently provides for new and important insights and perspectives. Simply attending events and becoming involved in groups can lead to future collaboration when this was not the original aim.

Within such groups we would also stress that you do some preparation and give some thought to the nature of the group and how you may be received within it:

It is important to know as much as you can about a group before endeavouring to network with the members. It is good to know the aims and objectives of the group, if possible, in advance. If a group represents a particular ethos then it is important to know and respect their position regardless of whether or not it fits in with yours. [Sheelah Flatman Watson]

What constraints do I face?

Additional to the issues of how you feel about networking and how to go about seeking out networking opportunities, further issues include how to fit networking into your research time-table. Some students can also experience several constraints limiting their networking opportunities. For example, other chapters in this volume illustrate the way family responsibilities and part-time studying can particularly limit the time and funding available for attending networking events. Accessing funding for opportunities may be difficult, but by taking a proactive approach some of our contributors found out about funding opportunities for research events and conferences. Childcare may be provided on request. Additional help at a conference with note-taking or accessibility may be available to those students with additional requirements, especially if you personally approach the organisers and can clearly specify your support needs. If you have a caring role and dependants you may not be able to attend as many conferences as you would like, but in being selective, using Web-based communication and looking widely for local opportunities, you may still be able to partake in several events. The stories of success that we have heard tended to come from students who weren't resigned to the constraints but took an active approach to seeking what was available and were strategic in networking.

BOX 8.3   Thinking about networking constraints

Think about what time you can put aside for attending events each semester and each year. Aiming to attend one major and one smaller event each year may be about right as you need to balance networking with the production of your thesis. Also seek out additional sources of support if you feel you need them. Many organisers of conferences and events are happy to work with you in ensuring you can participate. This will especially be the case if you approach them with plenty of time and some ideas. Additionally, some campaigning organisations, student unions or trusts may offer financial help for students to attend events.

Key Points to Remember

▶ Networking can have personal, social and professional benefits.
▶ Think through your assumptions and views of others working in your field of interest.
▶ Think through your approach and the value of networking.
▶ Attempt to map out networking opportunities by making a note of where authors are based, asking peers, asking supervisors and other academics, and researching the groups involved in all aspects of your field.
▶ Plan to attend key annual conferences and other seminar events in your field.
▶ Seek out opportunities beyond the academic setting.
▶ Think about what you can contribute to networks as well as what may be useful to you.
▶ Prepare before attending any event by finding out about the purpose, ethos and membership.
▶ Assess and review your experiences and keep a note of contact details.
▶ Think creatively, gain advice about and pursue ideas you have for establishing new networks.
▶ Be determined not to be excluded due to demands on you such as caring responsibilities – you have an equally valid and worthwhile role to play and ideas to contribute in your academic life, as well as having every right to be included and benefit!

SUGGESTED READING

Blaxter, L., Hughes, C. and Tight, M. (1998) *The Academic Career Handbook,* Buckingham: Open University Press.

Catt, H. and Scudamore, P. (2000) *30 Mins to Improve Your Networking Skills.* London: Kogan Page.

Grant, W. and Sherrington, P. (2006) *Managing Your Academic Career.* Basingstoke: Palgrave.

Phillips, M.P. and Pugh, D.S. (2005) *How to Get a PhD: A Handbook for Students and Their Supervisors*, 4th edn. Maidenhead Open University Press.

Wisker, G. (2001) *The Postgraduate Research Handbook.* Basingstoke: Palgrave.

Chapter 9

Missing the Deadline

- ▶ Submission rates and missing the deadline
- ▶ A lack of guidance and support
- ▶ Mismanaging the research process
- ▶ Personal circumstances
- ▶ Dealing with disappointment
- ▶ Enhancing the chances of meeting the deadline
- ▶ Setting deadlines and enhancing project management
- ▶ Voicing your concerns and seeking help

The broader picture: submission rates and missing the deadline

Until very recently, it remained the case that the majority of research students did not submit their thesis by the deadline stipulated by their funding council. A few years ago the average submission rates across the social sciences stood at 40% of research students submitting within four years if they were undertaking a PhD full-time with the remaining 60% of research students submitting later or not at all (Wright and Cochrane, 2000). Concerns have been raised about submission rates amongst research students in general, along with the particular concerns about the lower rates within the social sciences, and the need to re-structure doctoral research training. An over-arching theme arising from research undertaken on completion rates is that there are usually a combination of personal, institutional and method-ological factors leading to 'missing the deadline'. Research has recommended that universities should:

- Provide quality training in research methods and techniques.
- Monitor and standardise the quality of supervision.
- Evaluate student performance and progression throughout the PhD process.
- Provide a mixture of sanctions and incentives to encourage completion on time.
- Provide an extra (1+3) training year prior to doctoral study (Wright and Cochrane, 2000).

When studies have included student perspectives and experiences of 'missing the deadline', students attest to the following important contributing factors: feeling isolated, inadequate supervision and support, methodological problems and financial or personal difficulties during their doctoral studies (Becher et al., 1994; Hockey, 1994).

'Missing the deadline' is therefore a common student experience for many reasons. This chapter aims to recognise this common situation and consider some of the issues involved in students facing such a prospect. Ultimately, we hope to raise issues in order to prevent potential problems and enhance your chances of completing your PhD on time. If, however, 'missing the deadline' is something that occurs to you, we hope to provide some practical guidance and advice from other students who have lived through the experience! We will review some case studies that have particularly emphasised a lack of guidance and support, methodological or organisational problems and personal circumstances.

A lack of guidance and support

The overall message here seems to be problems with working out and negotiating the right kind of support, guidance and supervision at the right time. Different supervisors and universities can have alternative styles of supervision, which have emerged from alternative perspectives and traditions for supervising doctoral students towards successfully completing their studies on time (see Chapter 15). For example, a more traditional approach in the UK may be to allow a student a good measure of autonomy in confronting and coping with issues as they arise in their research studies. This may be viewed as the 'sink or swim' approach, or the best means through which to encourage the student to develop independence, academic authority or learning through experience. A more supportive and directive approach to supervision on the other hand may be viewed as either responsible supervision or 'encouraging dependency on the supervisor'. Phillips and Pugh (2005) note that in most cases supervisory relationships may move from a more directive towards a less directive approach as a student develops confidence and experience. However, several contributors to this book felt they suffered from either a lack of involved guidance and engagement from their supervisor, or inappropriate directive restrictions, leading to problems in setting and meeting deadlines:

> On [my supervisor's] return [following a year sabbatical during the second year of my thesis], it became apparent that he was not sensing my urgency and concerns for meeting the deadline. On one occasion he let slip that he thought I was in my second year of study. When I did submit some written work for him to look at, it

would take months to come back to me, often with very little feedback. We would meet on average every 2–3 months in the early stages, but this needed to change to every 2–3 weeks in Year 4. For whatever reason, this was not achievable. [Martin Smith]

Mismanaging the research process

With the benefit of hindsight and reflective thinking, several contributors to this book felt that they could have managed the research and doctoral process more efficiently and effectively. This illustrates the need to monitor and develop your methodological and research management skills. Collecting the right data for your study, allocating sufficient time for data collection and data analysis and establishing your findings are all processes that require considerable management during your studies. Additional to these general research processes are key aspects of PhD research – developing an argument, generating a thesis from your research and establishing an original contribution to a body of knowledge.

Martin Smith was surprised at the complexity of managing data collection, data analysis and the writing up process. He felt he had spent too much time on collecting data and not allowed enough time for data analysis and writing up. As we saw in Chapters 5 and 6, it is easy to get carried away with data collection and under-estimate the time required for data analysis and writing up. These research activities can also be very inter-related and can beneficially be viewed as connected processes as your findings and argument develop through cycles of engagement, analysis and thinking. Martin Smith spent over two years collecting data and then moved on to analysing and writing up. One difficulty that then arose, however, was the pressure of not having enough time to analyse or of having 'too much data'. Further, because Martin had collected the data without in-built checks on analysing the quality of the data, he also realised at a later stage that the data he collected was of 'poor quality':

I had collected a lot of information during the first three years of my PhD, but had very little to show in the way of written chapters. I had obtained more than 1,000 responses to a questionnaire and had inputted the data into a database for statistical

(Continued)

(Continued)

analysis. Alongside this, I had transcripts from focus groups. Whenever I spoke to my supervisor or colleagues about the quantity of information I had, they were generally impressed, although my supervisor was a little concerned that I should not try to do too much, and should not delay analysis and write-up any further. When it came to analysing the survey data, I found much missing data, vague responses and few patterns of interest. I found that the hypotheses I had set out to test could not readily be tested using my data. The focus group transcripts, too, did not produce the quality of material I needed to test my hypotheses. At this point, I had an urge to collect more data, but time was running out.

Such developments led to an increasing sense of concern and worry:

My difficulties began in the fourth and final year, when it came to 'the crunch', i.e. pulling the empirical data together; streamlining and organising my ideas to arrive at a 'thesis' or 'argument'; and producing a written thesis. Despite my best efforts, I simply could not write up the 'findings'. I felt I had little of interest to say, and felt that the points I was making were not tallying up to a bigger argument or overall verdict. It was due to inability to manage these tasks that I ended up missing the deadline and walking away from my PhD.
[Martin Smith]

Doug Morrison felt his approach to producing written work hampered his ability to meet deadlines throughout the PhD process. He felt he suffered from an excessive 'perfectionism':

As soon as I agreed to hand in a completed chapter, I became obsessed with handing in the perfect chapter. After all, this was my specialist area. I spent a long time rewording and rewriting. The consequence of this was handing in an either incomplete chapter or missing a deadline.

Being concerned with handing in a 'perfect chapter' can inhibit progress due to dissatisfaction with your work! In Chapter 6 we discussed the way writing can involve a process of formulating ideas through many drafts and further redrafting. Aiming for the 'perfect' chapter may well impede the progress of formulating your ideas as students become extremely critical of what are bound to be far from perfect early attempts at formulating an argument or writing up a chapter. If you are not happy with your initial attempts at writing chapters, we advocate that you value them as important first steps in a long process. Getting your ideas down, beginning to piece together the different aspects of your thesis and producing chapters at least in draft formats contribute to a sense that your thesis is developing and you are progressing towards the deadline. It may be worth attempting to value your first and second attempts at writing chapters and asking yourself if they are 'good enough' for now rather than 'perfect'. You may need to value the progressive steps towards improvement that you will need to take.

BOX 9.1   Techniques for project management and goal setting

A four-part approach to project management timetabling could include the following stages. Deadlines can be noted on sticky notes and then arranged onto a three-year timetable:

1   Work out and make a note of your major deadlines for each year of your research. These can be called milestones and may include your final submission deadline, second year upgrade, first year upgrade and final research proposal.
2   Break down each milestone into probable stages of work or steps towards reaching the milestone – for example, your final research proposal may include two weeks dedicated to each stage of the process including reviewing major literature; formulating research questions; thinking about your methods and design; thinking about ethics and writing up the proposal.
3   Arrange your tasks and milestones onto an annual or three-year timetable estimating the time required for each task. If all your tasks cannot fit in you will need then to re-think your activities and ask advice on whether you are estimating the time appropriately or attempting to do too much! Hopefully you will have over-estimated the time allowed to some degree, as you will need to allow for some deadlines to be missed or for the unexpected to occur!
4   Ask for advice from your supervisor on your milestones, tasks towards milestones and timetabling.

Personal circumstances

Circumstances such as the unexpected ill health of a relative or undertaking paid employment can hinder the progress towards meeting your submission deadline.

Martin Smith felt taking up full-time employment once his fourth year of funding ran out pulled him further away from the possibility of completing his PhD:

> As the end of the fourth year approached, I took a six-week long vacation. When I returned to the UK, I turned my attention to getting a full-time job. I was successful in getting a Research Officer post in the university. I had half a thesis in hand and a guaranteed income for the next 2 years. However, as I became more involved with my new job, I drifted further away from the PhD. The last thing I wanted to do on returning home in the evening was open up the thesis on the computer, or start analysing data. Weekends, too, were particularly hard. As each one came and went, I realised that I would not finish the thesis quickly, and it would in fact be harder than ever, especially as the remaining chapters would be the most challenging to produce.

Dealing with disappointment

Experiencing difficulties in meeting the submission deadline with time slipping away can be very demoralising. The combined feelings of worry, anxiety and insecurity can put even more pressure on a student at a time when extra effort and concentration is required to progress. Martin Smith found the final year of his PhD a time when increasing pressures and a fear of 'falling behind' compared to his peers contributed to a declining sense of self-pride, self-esteem and well-being. He describes a common process of 'losing pride in my work and confidence in myself'. He became 'very despondent' which in turn affected his relationships with others who 'became uneasy' around him. His confidence and motivation was further shaken as his peers started to complete their PhDs and move on.

A sense of falling behind can be very demoralising. Many students will be under pressure to complete within four years and will be concerned that their funding is also time-limited. Many can find dealing with such anxieties difficult, especially if other students appear to be progressing and even completing their research around you. While 'feeling the pressure' can be a spur to prioritise your studies and be more productive, long-term anxiety and stress can lead to emotional and physical exhaustion (see Chapters 14 and 18). The following sections consider some aspects of managing this situation and enhancing your progress towards overall deadline submission.

Enhancing the chances of meeting the deadline

Setting deadlines and enhancing project management

Your doctoral progress may be enhanced by analysing and developing your project management orientation and skills. It is unlikely that leaving the majority of the writing up to the last year will pay off as a strategy for completing a quality thesis. Project management is all about devising ways of mapping out the activities that make up your doctoral project and guiding your progress through a number of goals and stages. The idea is to break up your thesis into stages that are appropriate with realistic short-term and long-term deadlines that have been worked out and thought through in relation to the time available and objectives required. Setting targets can be part of a broader strategy of overall project management. This is about organising, monitoring and managing your progress throughout. At the very least the process will enhance your awareness of what can and needs to be done, and when. While project management does mean the 'what' and 'when' of your PhD are planned out, most approaches allow for flexibility and adjustment in the event of missed deadlines. A major benefit will be that any slippage is recognised at a very early stage and the whole 'project' can then be readjusted in line with new time constraints and deadlines. In planning out your research activities, you can break down your research project into major and minor milestones, thinking about long-term and short-term goals – a process detailed further in Box 9.1 above. You can also timetable in periods that you will need to dedicate to other commitments such as autumn semester teaching assistance or the family summer holiday.

Doug Morrison felt he could have benefited from more deadlines throughout his thesis as well as altering his approach. Such deadlines could have been viewed as helpful for monitoring and establishing progress rather than a demonstration of 'brilliance'. He reflects:

> In terms of material to be submitted, just remember that the purpose of the deadline is not to hand in a perfect piece of work. Indeed, with the benefit of hindsight, it is now clear that the main purpose of any deadline is to allow your supervisor to monitor your progress. Therefore, if you are unable to complete your work before the deadline, hand in what you have managed to do. This will allow your supervisor to monitor your progress, assess the cogency of your work and, as it progresses, the overall coherency of your thesis. Try to view the process as a means to an end rather than simply an end in itself.

BOX 9.2   Finding out about institutional regulations, doctoral milestones and submission regulations

Important information to find out about and inform your project timetable will be:

- University regulations for the submission of doctoral research.
- The timing and objectives of important progress milestones and assessments such as your annual report or MPhil upgrade submissions.
- Institutional policies on extensions for submissions and fees for additional years of study following the submission deadline.
- Timing for annual postgraduate conference or symposium events.
- Supervisory team expectations for deadlines for written work.
- Supervisory availability and absence from the university during your doctoral research.
- Procedures for supervision during supervisor absence.

Voicing your concerns and seeking help

You may need to proactively generate an approach akin to project management – encouraging your supervisor to set and negotiate a long-term perspective for deadlines throughout your thesis. If you start to get worried about your progress and feel you may be falling behind, a timetable approach will help you to spot any delays. Acting to re-schedule your timetable at the earliest possible stage may help you to avoid ultimately missing the submission deadline. However, for many reasons students delay 'speaking up' about their difficulties or worries:

If you are struggling to meet the deadline, whether due to writer's block, poor data quality or a difficult personal situation, do not be afraid to tell your supervisor. They are in a position, and have a responsibility, to assist you. Be direct with them. They should be able to look at your thesis plan and say what areas could be simplified, and what is less important. If you try to resolve these issues yourself, you run the risk of wasting precious time and making misguided choices. Let your supervisor take some of the responsibility, and change supervisors if you're not getting the support that you require. They might not be offended – they might be similarly relieved!
[Martin Smith]

Students may not want to draw attention to their difficulties, may not want to burden busy supervisors or appear too complaining. Struggling in silence, however, also does not seem to be a very effective way of overcoming problems in the PhD process:

> If some of your problems are personal ones, my advice is not to struggle on in silence as I did. Make an appointment with your supervisor and let them know what is going on. The deadline or deadlines can be re-arranged. You may even find that they have experienced similar situations themselves or have experience of such situations as a result of previous PhD candidates. In this scenario honesty is the best policy.
> [Doug Morrison]

What will be important is to find some way of thinking through your problems, concerns and options. If you prefer, this may involve writing your concerns and options down for yourself, and investigating what time and activities are required. However, there are many sources of support and accessing these resources could also be important for you in gaining advice and guidance that may help (see Part 4). Finding the right support and approaching a person with whom you feel at ease will be important.

Key Points to Remember

- ▶ Many research students submit their thesis in the year following their original deadline.
- ▶ Reasons for missing the deadline can vary and include inadequate supervision, over-ambitious research projects, lack of project management, methodological difficulties or personal/unexpected circumstances.
- ▶ Auditing and developing your project management and research management skills may help you to keep to schedule.
- ▶ Think about the role of your expectations and consider whether you are expecting too much or too little from yourself.
- ▶ Set long-term and short-term goals informed by your main yearly milestones throughout your project.
- ▶ Attempt to seek support and discuss your worries about meeting your deadline at an early stage and with your supervisor.

SUGGESTED READING

Dunleavy, P. (2003) *Authoring a PhD Thesis: How to Plan, Draft, Write and Finish a Doctoral Dissertation*. Basingstoke: Palgrave.

Howard, K., Sharp, J.A. and Peters, J. (eds) (2002) *The Management of a Student Research Project*. Aldershot: Gower.

Marshall, S. and Green, N. (2004) *Your PhD Companion*. Oxford: How To Books.

Tarling, R. (2005) *Managing Social Research*. London: Routledge.

Walliman, N.S.R. (2005) *Your Research Project: A Step-by-Step Guide for the First Time Researcher*. London: Sage.

Chapter 10
The Viva and Beyond

What this Chapter Includes:

▶ What happens after submission?
▶ How to prepare for the viva
▶ A brief look at the thesis examination
▶ An outline of the possible outcomes
▶ Tips for what to do in the post-viva stage
▶ Looking beyond the doctorate to getting a job
▶ Thinking about your career in tandem with writing up

You have submitted – now what?

After the thesis has been submitted there is an expectant period of waiting for the viva date. This can be filled with a mixture of either sheer relief, deep concern about the pending examination, or you may have reached the point of apathy. Hopefully, somewhere in your rainbow of emotions in the 'ending' stage you will still feel passionate for the topic and findings which should provide renewed enthusiasm for getting over the final hurdle. There are lots of different sources of information on how to prepare and succeed in the viva, as well as university and conference workshops and seminars that provide ample space to think and prepare for it. This chapter takes you through some of the basics with regard to planning and doing the examination, but we also look over the parapet at what happens afterwards. We think about planning the next career move during the writing up phase, as well as presenting some typical case scenarios of where and how doctorate social science and humanities students find jobs within the academy.

It may be of some comfort to know that there is much controversy amongst educationalists, university managers and academics regarding the place of the oral examination as the assessment form that judges the doctorate in the contemporary university setting. While the tradition of the oral defence of the thesis can be traced back to the Middle Ages, students now face a vastly different world of PhD study from 1917, when Oxford University imported the *viva voce* to Britain from the German system (Jackson and Tinkler, 2001: 356). Now, the concerns are with the need for transparency regarding the oral examination process, fairness, reliability and consistency within and across universities, resulting in a growing number of academics calling for a reform of this traditional system. Jackson and Tinkler (2001) conducted research to explore the purposes of the viva using university policy statements and the perspectives of academics and PhD candidates. This research concluded that there was 'no consensus regarding the roles of the viva in the PhD examination process' (2001: 66) and that there are substantial differences placed on the importance of the viva in the overall examination. While debates continue, students must work within the current regulations and the best way to do this is by understanding the process and preparing for the event from an early stage.

BOX 10.1   Check the regulations and administrative process in your institution

- What forms do you need to fill in before you submit?
- What criteria must be followed in terms of presentation and binding styles?
- Are there key dates when you can submit?

What we come to know about the 'viva' as a PhD student grows from academic mythology and legend that relays tales of students' dire experiences of being locked in an office for hours whilst subjected to an excruciating scrutiny of their work by two 'experts' who have used toothpicks to survey every sentence of the manuscript. The viva is tough and so it should be, given what is being awarded. It must be remembered that only a small percentage of students walk out of the viva with a 'no corrections' badge of approval as most students have work to complete and often have to resubmit the thesis after corrections have been made (see below). Moving away from the horror stories and positively framing the viva as an important stepping stone on the final home stretch can dispel myths and strangely help it become an event to look forward to. This is what this chapter hopes to do, and put you at ease about the examination process from the start.

The viva can be thought of as a special supervision session with two experts that can really shape what you do with your research findings and career. This may be the only time that you are 100% confident that all the people in the room have read, word for word, what you have written! The viva can be a meeting of minds, hopefully a discussion between intellectual equals – as, after all, you know your work better than anyone. (Just count how many times you are given that little gem of advice!) However, Gina Wisker is cautious:

> It is a mistake to think of the viva as a friendly chat among equals that will be quickly over, or equally to characterise it as a moment when the research can be presented as if at a conference. The viva offers a rare opportunity to share and deliberate over your work with experts but is also a strange mixture of a taxing and potentially exhilarating exchange.

The myths surrounding the viva are also fuelled by concerns about the role of the internal and external examiner and how they will perform when they are given the task of coming to an agreement over someone else's piece of work. Your PhD is in the firing line to become an intellectual battleground for academics who fiercely defend their territories and reputations! These competing dynamics mean that you should consider carefully who is approached to examine your thesis. Your supervisor, who also has a vested interest not to send you into a lion's den, usually guides this process. But choosing your examiners should be a joint decision that you are comfortable with.

How to prepare for the viva

The viva is like an unseen exam. You will not know the questions and the potential topics are broad. Preparing for the viva can also be conceptualised into two phases: long-term preparation and short-term revision. Like any exam preparation, the long-term planning takes the form of doing the work by attending the sessions and doing the reading, as well as a specific revision period before the exam. But first, let's see what criteria you need to fulfil in the viva.

Tinkler and Jackson (2004: 43) summarise what you are expected to do in the viva:

- Authenticate the thesis.
- Locate the research in the broader context.
- Clarify aspects of the thesis.
- Develop ideas.
- Justify aspects of the work.
- Reflect critically on the thesis.

This list of competencies may look daunting outlined here out of context, yet you should realise that this is what you have been doing in various ways throughout your PhD. Presenting your work, answering questions, relating your findings to the broader literature and critically reflecting and refining is what you will have done in your supervision sessions. Presenting at a conference or workshop, and passing various milestones such as upgrades are training opportunities in defending your work amongst peers and 'experts'.

BOX 10.2

Candidates should seek every opportunity to articulate and defend their work with others, explaining why they have chosen specific theories, methodology and methods, how the research question underpins all their research design and their argument, and how their work contributes to knowledge.
[Gina Wisker]

Long-term planning and preparation for the viva should be integrated into your progress. Engaging in the expected activities that require you to present your work will give you time to reflect on feedback, spruce up your communication skills and focus on how you conduct yourself when talking to others about your work.

Although preparation for the viva is an ongoing process, there are short-term revision tips that are helpful for when the thesis has been handed in. While preparation is important, time and space away from the manuscript is a crucial aspect of the reflection stage. Not picking up the thesis for a month after submission can be a relief, provide some distance from the emotions and stress of getting to submission and also enables some critical reflection to develop. Three weeks preparation time is a reasonable expectation. Here are some tips on how to approach the revision:

- Re-read the manuscript highlighting weaknesses, gaps and mistakes that are likely to be picked up by an examiner. Then prepare to be asked about these issues.
- Survey those who have recently gone through the viva experience – peer support is a must to dispel the grapevine horror stories.
- Take up the offer (or request one) of doing a mock viva with supervisors.
- Read the regulations and familiarise yourself with the possible outcomes.
- Be emotionally prepared – the viva is rarely the end.
- Think about the practicalities and arrangements on the day.
- Read a comprehensive study skills guide on how to prepare for the viva (see Suggested Reading).

Tinkler and Jackson (2004) have an excellent chapter dedicated to mock vivas that clearly sets out the advantages and limitations. Mock vivas can take several forms, including a video-taped format that you can take away and review, a peer audience of students, or a public mock viva where academics act out the scenario for others to learn from (2004: 138). Normally, your supervisor and another member of the department will conduct a mock viva with you to give you experience of the process. Hartley and Fox (2004) surveyed a small sample of students who underwent a mock viva and 90% (26) of respondents judged this form of preparation to be helpful. Mocks do steady the nerves, but like the real thing they still have to be prepared for and cannot be a complete likeness for the real one! If you undergo a mock viva, don't be complacent for the actual examination as it is most unlikely that the examiners will ask you the exact same questions.

BOX 10.3

It is important to rehearse how to frame, clarify, explore and express details of the thesis. Be prepared for questions that expect you to explain, describe and defend your work using the language of 'doctorateness' (words such as inductive, deductive, conceptual framework, theoretical perspectives, conceptual conclusions and so on).
[Gina Wisker]

As well as a long-and short-term preparation phase for the viva, Tinkler and Jackson (2004: 142) suggest a final stage of preparation in the days running up to the event. Their division of tasks between practical arrangements, meeting with your supervisor and academic preparations is a useful way of approaching those final couple of days before the examination.

The examination

When you are in the viva it is probably a fair assessment to say that it is a rather surreal experience. Your emotions and adrenalin are running high, as you feel it is the most important day of your life and that the two people sitting in front of you have your future pathway at their fingertips. Do not under-estimate the power of nerves and take precautions to address these. Wear comfortable clothing, but remember also this is a formal occasion. Drink to ensure you are well hydrated and take deep breaths. Take a copy of the thesis with you and don't be alarmed when you see hundreds of sticky notes sticking out of the examiners' copies. Remember to take notes and ask questions from the examiners. Use affirmative language that qualifies your piece of work as original, robust and contributing new knowledge to the field. Have a tick list of areas that you are particularly keen to talk about and make sure you bring the discussion round to including these. At the end of the viva be very clear about what the examiners are recommending and their specific advice. Ask the examiners to go through what happens next.

It is very important to be prepared for the outcome. The examiners have four options to choose from when considering their recommendation. You should consult your institution's own guidelines but the basic outcomes are:

- Award with no corrections
- Award subject to minor corrections
- Referral
- No award or award at a lower degree

All of these outcomes have various details, criteria and timescales attached which you should find out about nearer to the time. You will be sent an examiners' report that is the formal record of the event with some clear pointers for change. Remember, if you fail the viva and you think there are mitigating circumstances (such as the university's procedures were not followed, the examination panel was inappropriate or personality clashes) then there is a robust appeals process.

Post viva: celebration, commiseration and more work!

It is a misconception that the PhD is finished at the viva stage. It is true that a thesis should only be submitted for examination if the supervisor and student feel that the work is at the necessary standard, but usually there is further work to be done, which could be anything from a few typos and grammar corrections to a substantial rewrite. Gina Wisker suggests that how students think about the viva can prepare them for the realistic likelihood that there will be more work to be done afterwards:

Most PhD students and supervisors view the viva as the last part of the PhD process. But with so few PhDs actually being awarded with absolutely no corrections, it can actually be more realistically seen as a major moment of summative assessment which acts as one of formative assessment and feedback, leading to revisions and the strengthening of the PhD.

Sonali Shah submitted her PhD in the social sciences after four years and was at a loss to find out this was not the end:

I was so relieved and excited when I saw all seven chapters of my work printed and bound together that I never imagined the end was not yet in full view. The end was, in actual fact, another year away, which I discovered after spending two hours trying to defend my thesis to a couple of strangers, only to get referred and be given another year to rewrite the whole thing before resubmission.

There can clearly be a range of outcomes from the viva that mean different types of work are required. But whether you are referred or pass without corrections, there will still be work to be done. The formula for learning from the viva does not only rest in the final examiners' report, but alongside your supervisor you should reflect on what was said in the viva and make a list of the advice and tasks based on short-, medium- and long-term changes. Gina Wisker reflects on a case where the student was referred, and demonstrates a useful strategy for learning from the examiners and taking an action plan forward:

Together with the supervisor the student reviewed the recommendations of the examiners, turning these into an agenda for the new work that would make more use of the research question, argument and the data. A revised timeline, some targets and serious discussions about the elements of the thesis that required clarity and conceptual work supported this agenda.

If you are one of the few that has passed with flying colours then there are questions about how to take the thesis forward. Should it be turned into a book and therefore requiring a book proposal and the search for a publisher? Or, how many articles can be extracted from the thesis, for which journals and in what order of priority? Do I have obligations to disseminate my work to the participants, users, gatekeepers and policymakers? If, like many, you have minor corrections to make, what is the timescale for these and how will they be actioned given your current work commitments? Either way, the outcomes of the viva inevitably mean that there is more work to be done before being awarded the doctorate or to achieve the next career move.

Thinking about 'after' before it arrives

Obviously it is not the case that PhD students begin to consider their careers after the viva or when the doctorate is finally awarded. Recalling the motivations for starting a PhD outlined in Chapter 1, it is clear that many students are very focused on their career pathways from day one. This section therefore will highlight some key tips for thinking about getting a job whilst still working towards the PhD and how various milestones can be met before you are actually ready to send off applications.

There are several long-term activities that can help build momentum for your next step after the PhD. Justin Waring was convinced he wanted to stay in academia from an early stage, so began arming himself with knowledge of the job market while he was writing up the thesis:

Through attending seminars such as University Research Training modules in 'CV Writing' and 'Interview Skills' together with searching career websites I was informed about the many avenues and opportunities for progression. The options ranged from post-doctoral studentships, early career fellowships or research grants, to teaching or research appointments. I sought out other opportunities, through making almost daily searches of *jobs.ac.uk* and never missed Tuesday's *Guardian*.

There are several options for the student who wants to continue with their research and teaching interests, some of which Justin outlines above. However, the criteria for entering into academia in this particular climate of the Research Assessment Exercise, the emphasis on winning research money and publications is daunting for those just starting out. Justin explains how he slowly realised that the criterion for entering academia is not only the award of a doctorate; other badges of proof are required.

Exposure to the job market highlighted a further important issue for career progression: the need to write from my work, either as a monograph or in peer reviewed journals, to further prove the intellectual worth of my studies to the outside world. I was fully aware that the development of a 'publication profile' goes hand-in-hand with post-doctoral progression: the idea of 'publish or die' is firmly established in academic parlance.

BOX 10.6 Build up your CV

If you want a career in academia it is important to build up your CV over time, aiming to include some publications before you apply for post-doctoral employment. Teaching experience is also important if you want to apply for a lectureship.

One of the familiar steps into 'the academy' is to take up work as a contract researcher. Despite this being an embedded aspect of the research culture, little is written about this type of work. Collinson (2003) has written about the marginal status of the contract researcher, and although employment rights have been strengthened recently, this job is fraught with instability because contracts rarely go beyond two years. Justin Waring took up contract research and reflects on the negative aspects:

In the academic world I have found nothing quite as demoralising, depressing and in many ways disrespectful to the hard work of a researcher than the short-term and insecure nature of contract research.

The inherent nature of short–term contract work is usually what PhD students want to avoid after a fairly unorthodox period of several years with a minimum salary and obvious financial worries. But there are clear benefits of doing contract research:

- Working on a new topic and new data.
- Using new and alternative methodology.
- Developing your own topic.
- Extending networks.
- Time for writing papers and teaching.
- Developing your CV and specific research training.

Contract research work is often a viable stop-gap whilst finishing off the doctorate or look-ing for permanent employment. Make sure you are clear what your contract includes and negotiate time for writing up papers from your doctorate and early career development. How will the contract research job benefit you?

There are other wider structural issues to consider when choosing a career in academia. Finch (2003: 133) describes how the organisational environment of universities also reflects both the horizontal and vertical gender segregation of women's position in the labour market. Finch reports that in pre-1992 universities women occupy less than one-quarter of academic posts while the proportion of female professorships remains on average 10%. Rangasamy (2004) provides research that identifies four aspects of institutional racism in Higher Education: the legacy of colonial thinking; active discrimination; conservatism and institutional defensiveness. Universities are old, white, male institutions and while interventions to do something about institutional racism are under way, the reproduction of racism through the 'sheer weight of white-ness' (Back, 2004: 1) will take a while to unpick. While not wanting to disillusion students, it must be remembered that although academia is quite different from many other employment sectors, the inequalities and segregation that exist in society are not exempt from university settings.

Non-academic careers

Of course, PhD students do not necessarily stay in academia. Figures show that in 2003 (UK Grad Programme, 2004: 14–15), the 3,765 UK-domiciled PhD graduates working in the UK were spread across a range of employment sectors:

- 16% worked in manufacturing
- 16% worked in health and social care
- 9% worked in finance and IT sector
- 6% worked in public administration
- 48% worked in education

There are two ways of considering applying your PhD outside academia:

1   Using your knowledge to enter a specialist field that will utilise:

- Scientific research knowledge
- Expert knowledge in a particular subject
- Specific research skills

- Policy knowledge and development skills
- Working with particular user groups, communities and social issues

2   Opting for an unconnected professional career that will:

- Utilise your broader project management skills
- Use researcher skills for unrelated areas
- Apply problem-solving and analytical skills
- Enhance communication, written and oral skills

Such professions include management consultancy, investment banking, professional services and public administration. Many of the large multinational companies seek people with a PhD to take on management roles that require generic training to a high standard. PhD graduates with skills in quantitative methods are directly sought by investment banking companies.

BOX 10.8   Non-academic careers

UK Grad Programme offers lots of information for non-academic careers. Check out the GRAD Schools and the Careers in Focus programme, which is free and will benefit you in the following ways:

- Meet people currently working in other professions
- Hear about the job in detail
- Learn about the application process
- Ask questions that are specific to your circumstances
- Learn about the working environment

One important thing to remember is that you have acquired a critical and analytical mind, with self-motivation and the ability to work autonomously on a large project. These are skills that are marketable, so whether you are inside or outside academia, you have a lot to offer employers.

BOX 10.9

Doctorate graduates are the most highly skilled and educated group produced by the British education system, so be mindful of your specialist transferable skills, which many different employment sectors will be attracted to.

▶ Preparing to defend your thesis and proficiently answer questions about your work should be weaved into your overall progress and not just something to think about preparing before the viva.

▶ Preparation can be conceptualised as long-term, short-term revision and the final stages.

▶ Do your research and discuss with your supervisor who are the best examiners. You should have considerable input here.

▶ There are four outcomes that examiners can recommend – be clear what they mean.

▶ The viva is not the symbolic ending of the PhD that legend would have it. Whatever the recommendation, it will mean more work.

▶ If looking for a career in academia and research, attention should be given to what is expected, in particular peer reviewed publications, early on in your career planning.

▶ Institutional racism and gender segregation in Higher Education do not make academia any more protected from structural inequalities than other sectors.

SUGGESTED READING AND RESOURCES

Murray, R. (2003) *How to Survive Your Viva: Defending a Thesis in an Oral Examination.* Maidenhead: Open University Press.

Secrist, J. and Fitzpatrick, J. (2000) *What Else You Can Do With a PhD.* London: Sage.

Tinkler, P. and Jackson, C. (2004) *The Doctoral Examination Process.* Maidenhead: Open University Press.

Part III
Shifting Identities and Institutions

In this third section we wanted to take a fresh look at the people who are taking doctoral studies in the contemporary academic setting and how their identities were affected by the processes of doing a PhD. In this section, we focus on how students' identities are affected by studying and working towards a PhD. They are changed by taking on new roles and working with old roles and experiences. Not only will you come out of the doctorate having produced an original piece of work, but no doubt you will have done a lot of work on yourself in the meantime.

Long gone is the pattern where students move from undergraduate to masters and then PhD studies in a succinct, continuous flow. Often PhD studies are taken in conjunction with work commitments, after a career, alongside a career and frequently with family commitments to bear in mind. We start this section of the book with Chapter 11 reflecting on how people come into PhD study from different routes, highlighting that the non-traditional route could fast become the dominant entrance route into postgraduate study. Taking on a PhD later in the lifecourse brings with it additional issues that are important to consider as everyday occurrences for those entering education at a later stage. Here we deal with the rub between work experience and entering a world of study that can seem very alienating. We make links between skills and tasks often performed in other work environments to identify core transferable skills. Equally we look at the rise in 'professional doctorates' as an option for those professionals already involved in career trajectories.

Increasingly, students are taking on PhDs on a part-time basis. We considered this to be a growing area that warranted a specific look at the pros and cons of studying part-time. Here, specific issues such as time management and being away from the institution for the majority of time are looked at from the student's perspective. Chapter 13 takes a look at the relationship between doing teaching work whilst continuing with the research degree. Teaching undergraduates when doing your doctorate is a very common experience, yet receives little consideration from the student's viewpoint. We look at the benefits for taking on teaching, how to protect your research time and corner-cutting strategies to save you a few extra hours in the week when preparing for teaching. Chapter 14 puts the emotional aspect of doing a PhD into the spotlight. Taking on board this task is an emotional journey and our contributors reflect on how their emotions were implicated both in doing the research and also doing the PhD as separate but interlinked processes.

Chapter 11
Non-traditional Routes into the PhD

What this Chapter Includes:

- ▶ Alternative routes into doctoral studies
- ▶ Special issues for older postgraduates
- ▶ Adapting to a new way of working
- ▶ Applying previous experience to new challenges
- ▶ The complexities of managing several identities
- ▶ The differences and similarities between work and research
- ▶ Professional doctorates

Starting a PhD later in the lifecourse

The changing nature of Higher Education and the workplace in the twenty-first Century now means that it is no longer the case that the majority of PhD students are those who have traditionally come straight from an undergraduate degree (also see Chapter 16). The most common path is to take an MA or to work in various related and unrelated work settings before contemplating a PhD. With a rise in distance learning postgraduate courses from diplomas, certificates, masters level courses as well as a few universities offering PhDs on a distance learning basis, studying is taking on new and innovative forms. Distance learning courses are a popular avenue to re-entering education and gaining a qualification without making geographical changes. The competition for funding is now so fierce that successful candidates often already have a postgraduate qualification and/or experience from a career before applying. The last ten years have seen a rise in the number of non-traditional routes into doctoral education as individuals are presented with opportunities to undergo independent study at a later stage in the lifecourse. As noted in Chapter 1, the reasons for taking on doctoral studies can be to develop an existing career or can be a gateway into a new career. Whatever the motivations, for older people returning to Higher Education there are some specific issues to consider and practical suggestions for tackling unfamiliar ground. This chapter looks at the experiences of mature students, their transition from other jobs to doing a doctorate, and offers some strategies to help the transition go smoothly.

Older students – returning to study

Whatever the domestic circumstances, the decision to re-enter Higher Education is not taken lightly by those who are returning to education after 'a life elsewhere'. Osborne, Marks and Turner (2004) conducted a large-scale study exploring the decision making of mature students to return to education. They found a typology of six different categories of people:

- Delayed traditional students.
- Late starters.
- Single parents.
- Careerists.
- Escapees.
- Personal growers.

These categories highlight distinct motivating factors that may encourage people to re-enter education, while at the same time the categories reinforce how older students are taking on study often under very different circumstances to their younger peers.

Melanie Shearn reflects on her contemplation of doing a PhD whilst having a family and leaving a career.

> There were two main factors that concerned me while I considered applying for a PhD. Could I afford it, and could I stick out three years working on one project by myself? Could I go back to being a full-time student for that period of time?

Someone who has re-entered education at a later stage will face complex dynamics of juggling other roles and commitments whilst starting out on a new path. This can produce both anxiety and exhilaration, but inevitably becoming a 'mature' student means taking on additional roles. Bill Armer re-entered education in his 40s and went on to complete a PhD in 2005. Here, he reflects on the issue of juggling identities and recognises that as an older person there is more at stake:

As an older person, you are likely to carry far more labels – perhaps parent, carer, provider, partner – than your 'standard' colleagues. This means that you will not usually be categorised as simply 'a student'. The unifying factor is that 'responsibility' very often translates into monetary need, and almost always infers an emotional tug of war between the competing demands of 'significant others' on our time and energy and our own desire for personal (and perhaps financial) fulfilment.

Remembering that Higher Education has traditionally been the domain for the white male middle classes, there are tensions here between the relationships of class, ethnicity and gender in the traditional Higher Education settings. Marks (2003) explains the historical traditions of the ambivalent relationship between working class men and Higher Education while Britton and Baxter (1999) note that becoming a mature student has different meanings for men and women. Older students often carry more personal and familial commitments than the traditional doctorate student who is under 30 years old and often with fewer life commitments. While the majority of older students may have family commitments, women with children will undoubtedly be faced with a double burden of both caring commitments and managing a household as well as studying and/or employment (Raddon, 2002). Care commitments to children and elders often feature as a significant compromise for female older PhD students as their studies are often affected by circumstances outside their control. The double burdens that women in academia may feel are compounded by a patriarchal institution that has been built on a sharp gender divide resulting in women facing different challenges to men in doctoral studies (Kurtz-Costes et al., 2006). Life commitments have implications for how the game is played and the type of 'studenthood' that is experienced. These additional tensions relating to gender, class and age may well play out in the decision to put your hand up for the demanding job of juggling a work–life balance with a programme of research that has fluid boundaries and somewhat unconventional demands.

BOX 11.1   Female doctoral students

Female students, especially those with care commitments, may have a different experience from male peers due to the historical gender imbalance that university systems are built upon. Check for instance about flexible working hours, if meetings can be in school hours, the balance of women in the Faculty, the provisions for childcare from your funders etc. (also see Chapter 17).

Alongside gender, age is invariably a social factor that influences the experiences of older students. You may well encounter negative images and treatment as a result of ageism and discrimination may not be directly obvious. Older students can often feel pressure to demonstrate their wisdom and knowledge gained through work and life experience. This can lead to older students not being given the same attention as younger students because there is an assumption that they can cope. In a world where technology shapes our lives, an area of tension can be that of technology and computing. Many IT skills, such as emailing and using Microsoft Word, are now considered life skills that are acquired outside the university setting and therefore it is assumed that all students already have this capability. It may be that as an older student the technological revolution has passed you by and you are not as technologically equipped as the course organisers assume. This demonstrates how some older students feel the university setting is predicated on 'assumptions of competence' (Phillips and Pugh, 2005: 129), which ignores the situation that older students often find themselves in. A lack of understanding from the university system that some students do not come from traditional routes can breed feelings of resistance and resentment. Below we analyse how the PhD can be approached as if it were a job, transferring strategies from mainstream employment to tackle the unwieldy and vague reality of doing a PhD.

Applying work wisdom to the challenge of academia

Moving out of a full-time career back into the unfamiliarity of Higher Education can be an anxious change. Returning to education after a 'life elsewhere' can be an advantage as a wealth of experience gained in other jobs can be effectively applied to doctoral studies from the outset. Managing a previous career has invariably meant working to deadlines, project management and timetabling, co-operating and negotiating with line managers, finding solutions to complex problems, working autonomously, being resourceful and making and sustaining new networks. All these skills are entirely transferable, and indeed very useful, to the PhD.

A strong theme that came out of speaking with postgraduates about approaches or 'philosophies' for approaching the PhD was to consider the research project like a job:

> Put simply, the important thing to do is to consider the research programme as a job. Poorly paid, but intrinsically interesting and offering the real potential of career advancement.
> [Bill Armer]

> The approach I've taken with my PhD is to treat it like a job. My 'jobs' in the past have been in the private sector and have always involved very tight deadlines to which I would be held accountable.
> [Melanie Shearn]

All of the students we spoke to while writing this book described how skills and strategies that they had learnt from other environments could be adapted to the PhD experience. This was often related to managing tight deadlines, working in teams, collaborating with others, presenting material and time management. Richard Heslop, who is studying for a doctorate in education whilst maintaining his job as a full-time police officer, reflects on how the two jobs are not that dissimilar:

> As a police officer I have always had to be organised and methodical in my work. In terms of my research methodology (interviews), police work certainly gives me the interpersonal and questioning skills to make the work easier.

Richard found that alongside specific transferable skills, such as interview techniques, problem-solving was often a key skill that could be applied to the PhD process that made the current job much less stressful. Melanie Shearn found that being able to troubleshoot and work through problems made the light at the end of the tunnel always visible rather than sitting in the dark for days, contemplating a difficulty that generates only procrastination:

> The jobs I previously held required a lot of multi-tasking, problem solving and short deadlines. As a result I think I am far more organised now and my project and time management skills are much more advanced ... Research problems for me are just blips that I cope with far better than I would have before my work experience.

Often these skills are embedded in the way in which we approach tasks, understand objectives and set out a path to achieve them. The transference of skills may be both conscious and unconscious, but be assured that if you are approaching postgraduate study from a non-traditional route, then you will be bringing useful skills, strategies and stress-busting techniques.

BOX 11.2

As with any other job, there are four major factors to consider with the PhD: pay, duties, hours of work and job satisfaction. Consider these carefully before committing yourself to a course of study, and involve your significant others in the deliberations. [Bill Armer]

Starting a PhD after a lengthy career elsewhere can also bring with it conflicts of interests and it may take a while for one role to be replaced by another. Ruth Bartlett was awarded a case studentship (joint funding from a research council and another body – in this case the ESRC and a large charitable housing organisation) after she had spent many years as a mental health nurse working with people with dementia. Ruth's PhD was still to be in this area but she was now in the role of 'researcher' and not 'nurse', which turned out to be a complex and somewhat difficult change. Ruth explains why:

> As a nurse with clinical experience of working with people with dementia, in a research environment I found myself reflecting upon my motives and position as a doctoral researcher very early on in the study …. Having been trained to help people with this condition in a very practical and often immediate way, some of the comments participants made to me during the study, such as 'so you're here to help yourself then, not me', cause me to reflect upon and question the utility of qualitative research, particularly when undertaken by doctoral students.

Shifts in identity are part of the process of moving into the researcher role and, as Ruth experienced, this can flag up some difficult issues both emotionally and practically.

It's work, but not as you know It: recognising the differences

While we want to emphasise the transferable skills that all students will have, we also want to give a realistic perspective on the differences that students coming back into Higher Education will face with the PhD project. The PhD can be treated like a job in terms of how your day is structured, recognising the funding as a salary, and treating supervisors as line managers who are there to guide your project to success. Yet there are still some intrinsic differences between mainstream work and doing a PhD because of the nature of original and independent research. Melanie Shearn reflects on the similarities and differences between mainstream employment and research work:

> While my funding helps to give me the feeling that my PhD's a job, and my background in freelancing means I'm used to working from home, there are downsides to treating it like a job. For starters, it's far more isolating than any job I've ever had. Even when I freelanced, I had contact with people who had a stake in the project. During my PhD, I've found that there is nobody working on my PhD except me – and I don't like that: to whom am I accountable and in what way?

The isolation and loneliness that students often feel is a familiar feature of doctoral studies. This is in marked contrast to many other work settings where the emphasis is on team work, or even if individual autonomy and responsibility is common, it is rarely the case to the extent it is with doctoral work that you are the sole individual responsible for producing everything! With a PhD, the weightiness of responsibility that the buck stops with you can be overwhelming. Melanie goes on to offer suggestions for managing feelings of isolation:

> One of the most useful things I've found in terms of 'connecting' both my project and myself to the world is to build up a network of contacts with people working on similar projects at other universities.

Remember that PhD topics are so specific that it is unlikely another student will be doing an exactly similar area. This can increase feelings of isolation and highlights why networking outside your institution is crucial.

BOX 11.3

Chapter 8 on 'Networking' provides strategies to deal with the isolating consequences of independent study while Chapter 16 discusses how challenging environments can be tackled.

No doubt moving out of the workplace, or even reducing full-time hours to take on a PhD part-time, will be met with jokes and jibes from colleagues and family about how students spend hours over coffee breaks, musing in academic circles and gently perusing the library shelves for inspiration! These are grossly inflated stereotypes (well, 99%) as the reality of completing a huge piece of work in three years becomes clear. Time is not a luxury in doctoral studies. Bill Armer has some words of warning about how to manage time:

> Don't fall into the trap of muttering to yourself 'I've got another three years to catch up' – time has a habit of eluding you. As far as possible treat your studies as a job with a set number of hours of weekly work. Arrange a programme that suits you and your lifestyle, but aim to work for about thirty hours a week (on a full-time basis) in manageable blocks. An hour is probably too short to be useful, four hours may well test your concentration to its limit or beyond. Know yourself and be realistic, but don't forget that, in this context, 'work' may consist of reading, quiet contemplation or writing-up.

The nature of research work and what it actually means to 'write a PhD' can be elusive to those doing it, let alone to those who are on the periphery peering into the unknown world of being a PhD student. The reality will be that even when working from home, which is a popular option these days as sometimes the environment is preferable, those around need to be aware that you are in 'DO NOT DISTURB' mode. Bill Armer explains how doing a PhD in a home environment has implications for those who share your home:

> Partners, children and any others who depend upon you for support will need to accept that, just as if you had a 'real' job, there will be times when you are not available except in an emergency. You might be 'only' reading a book, or even just quietly thinking, but impress upon them that you are not to be disturbed.

Thinking time is something that is important at all stages of the PhD, whether it be when designing the methodology, reflecting on fieldwork or contemplating your findings and developing new concepts.

Professional doctorates

There is little publicity about the non-traditional routes into doctorate education and the opportunities of undertaking postgraduate study in the form of a professional doctorate. Although not available in all UK universities, this system was imported from North America in 1992 and is favoured by disciplines and professions that are practice-based. It is known to challenge traditional formats of the PhD because it is 'explicitly concerned with practical knowing and doing' (Lester, 2004: 762). For instance, nursing (D.Nursing), social work (D.S.W.), education (Ed.D), medicine (MD), engineering (EngD) and clinical psychology (DClinPsychol) are more familiar paths for clinicians and practitioners. At least 38 of 70 UK universities surveyed offer at least one professional doctorate programme across 19 disciplines (Bourner et al., 2001: 67).

Known also as 'practitioner doctorates' (Lester, 2004: 757), these programmes offer a general emphasis on a combination of taught courses, practice, research training and original research, which includes a thesis of around 40,000 words (somewhat shorter than the traditional thesis length which is around 80,000). These independent pieces of research emerged from 'the contexts of the academy, the profession and the workplace or practicum' (Lester, 2004: 758). The requirement to demonstrate independent and critical thinking as well as make a contribution to the academic field is at the same standard as a traditional doctorate. In no way is doing a professional doctorate a lighter option compared to the traditional route! In fact the professional doctorate has grown in popularity amongst university managers and educational reformists as well as students because of the deficiencies in the traditional doctorate pathway that neither reflects the reality of those working in practice professions but offers a more contemporary approach to learning and knowledge production.

The modern day approach of the professional doctorate can suit students who are still pursuing regular jobs and combining their postgraduate studies with the demands of everyday employment. Richard Heslop has pursued Higher Education for the past ten years alongside full-time employment in the police force. After gaining an undergraduate degree from the Open University in politics followed by a masters and a PGCE, his new position as a police trainer developed his interest in adult education. This led to his enrolment on a Doctor of Education programme on a part-time basis. Richard explains the benefits of this route:

> There were a number of advantages for taking the EdD over a traditional PhD. In large part this was to do with the structured modular approach of the programme … During the first two and a half years of my EdD I was required to complete five taught 'specialist' modules from relevant masters programmes, across the university, two had to be on research methodology. This gave me ample opportunity to mix with and bounce my ideas off other students in the early stages of the degree.

The taught elements of the professional doctorate can help combat some of the perennial problems associated with independent study. Loneliness and isolation are most easily dealt with through networking, working in small groups and sharing ideas about research and practice. The professional doctorate specifically addresses these difficulties providing a productive learning environment that fosters peer support.

Key Points to Remember

▶ Non-traditional routes in doctoral education are increasing as more older students enter Higher Education.

▶ Alongside age, there are particular dynamics in relation to gender, class and ethnicity for students, so make sure you seek out advice networks and others in similar situations.

▶ Achieving a work-life balance is crucial if there are other people whom you have responsibilities for. This is a point for discussion and action pre-enrolment!

▶ Experience, skills and strategies gained from previous employment are vital and can be transferred to managing the PhD.

- The PhD can be structured like a job with set hours and a familiar work structure.
- The professional doctorate is a good option for those in specific practitioner-based occupations.

SUGGESTED READING

Becker, L. (2004) *How to Manage Your Distance and Open Learning Course*. Basingstoke: Palgrave.

Burgess, H., Slemnski, S. and Arthur, L. (2006) *Achieving Your Doctorate in Education*. London: Sage.

Green, B., Maxwell, T.W. and Shananhan, P.J. (eds) (2001) *Doctoral Education and Professional Practice*. Armidale, NSW: Kardoorair Press.

Powell, S. (2001) *Returning to Study*. Buckingham: Open University Press.

Rose, J. (2001) *The Mature Student's Guide to Writing*. London: Palgrave.

Scott, D. (2004) *Professional Doctorates: Integrating Academic and Professional Knowledge*. Maidenhead: Open University Press.

Chapter 12
Undertaking a PhD Part-time

What this Chapter Includes:

▶ Explorations of why this is a viable route
▶ Questions to consider before signing up
▶ The reality of doing a job and studying
▶ Tips for prioritising study
▶ Overview of competencies for postgraduate study
▶ Time management strategies

Why part-time study?

Largely thanks to pioneers such as the Open University, which offers flexible Higher Education to those who want to combine studies with other commitments, it is possible to study for a doctorate on a part-time basis. The Open University is renowned for its flexibility as its ethos was built on distance learning. Making optimal use of computer technology through e-learning websites and modes of communication, there are many MA level distance courses that can be taken on a full- or part-time basis across universities in the UK. In more recent years, most universities have recognised that part-time study is attractive to a proportion of postgraduate students and offer a system to accommodate this. In some disciplines, especially professional doctorates, part-time students are the majority. Part-time students are generally combining the research with a full-time paid job or a full-time care commitment. It may be that studying and working simultaneously is the right choice for you, either due to finances or because your everyday work informs your research agenda. It may be that the PhD is part of continuing professional development and that it is an extension of work rather than a separate entity. Either way, the part-time route presents different obstacles than the full-time route as, after all, the doctorate system is very much geared up to the four-year full-time completion rate (including one year's formal training). However, do not be put off. Claire Maxwell finished her PhD part-time in just over five years and fully recommends combining work and independent research:

There is no doubt that doing a PhD part-time is more challenging than doing one full-time. But everyone has other commitments and responsibilities, so the same principles apply to finding the right balance between completing your PhD while meeting your other responsibilities. Despite the challenges, I don't regret doing my PhD part-time because it meant I developed my career at the same time, and, very importantly, I think working also kept me sane!

It is often wise to connect your PhD topic to your everyday job because it makes life easier. Often resources can be used from work, gatekeepers and access to research participants are easier because of your 'insider' status (don't forget there are ethical issues with this as well), and occasionally the research can be done in work time. For example, contributors to this book who studied part-time closely aligned their topic with their day job. Sallyann Halliday worked as a researcher and decided to study the contract research culture as an occupation; Richard Heslop was a trainer in the police service and opted to study the relationship between police training and adult education. Claire Maxwell was a social worker and went on to explore young people's sexual relationships. These choices make sense because there were continuities between full-time work and part-time study.

Taking the plunge!

The motivations to do a PhD are similar for part-time as they are for full-time students (see Chapter 1). Yet, often the decision to enrol and actually 'take the plunge' is the result of lots of queries and quibbles, angst and self-doubt. Sallyann Halliday had studied for a masters part-time so was aware of the juggling act between work and study. Yet her contemplation of doing a PhD brought renewed concerns about how she would actually fit the study in:

There were so many concerns and thoughts going through my head, such as – How would I fit PhD study in? Would my employer pay for it and support me? Would I be given study leave? Actually how, in practical day-to-day, 'get real' terms, I would fit it in with a busy full-time job was a worry at first. In my mind, making sure I could balance the demands of the duties of my full-time professional position alongside the demands of part-time doctoral study was important.

Realistically weighing up how you will squeeze this additional commitment into your already full schedule has to be the first reality check. Frank discussions with those at home and your employer are essential before you decide to take this task onboard. If you will get no 'help', whether this is financial, study leave or resources from your employer, then perhaps this is not the right time to take on board the challenge. Sallyann Halliday recounts how confronting her boss was a useful step in the decision making to undertake a PhD part-time whilst still working, and was lucky to receive full support:

> When I decided that I was going to undertake a PhD, I arranged a meeting with my boss to discuss with him how I would like to carry on with part-time study as well as my full-time position. I received their full support in the form of payment of fees and study leave. My boss, a Professor, was encouraging and gave wise words of advice to me, most notably 'it's hard work – but worth it'.

You may not work in such a sympathetic work culture but instead one where doctorates are not the ordinary pathway. This may mean your negotiations are more complex and will need thinking through.

What is important is not to have unrealistic expectations of what PhD study will be like. Universities are traditional institutions, built on old-fashioned stereotypes of students. Although the new universities (post 1992) will have some different approaches to the student experience, teaching, research priorities and general philosophies, the older universities are set up very traditionally. Some of the contributors talked of a 'culture shock' when they began postgraduate study because the research culture was a rather different culture to mainstream employment. For instance, referring to her other employment experience, an older student and also a mother, Melanie Shearn offers her observations on how university can have its own peculiar approach:

> Coming to do my PhD at a university that caters for more 'traditional' work hours and people aged around 18–21 was a bit of a culture shock. I have found that my experiences, interests and time schedules form barriers to participation in some activities. I also find the student–staff relationship trickier because I'm closer in age to some of the younger staff.

Many part-time doctoral students have done part-time study before. Remember that a PhD will not be a short period of cramming that you may be familiar with after doing a dissertation. This is a commitment that will last six years! You must be ready for the long run.

Obvious hurdles

The experiences that part-time PhD students face are often similar to those that full-time students experience. Concerns that have been outlined throughout the book are all applicable to the part-time student. But there are some peculiarities that are specifically related to part-time status. Below we discuss some of the more obvious issues that manifest for the part-time student.

Out on a limb

Being part-time ultimately means you spend less of your working week engaged with the institution, the work or in contact with peers in the working environment. This may lead to feelings of displacement: that you are attached to the department but you are removed by the limited amount of time you spend there. This can lead to uncertainties about what you are actually meant to be doing, as you have fewer indicators around you from peers and therefore no benchmarks for comparison. Below, Sallyann Halliday reflects on how she was a little confused about the amount of work she should be doing as she had no likeminded peer with whom she could assess the pace of her work:

> When I first started, I was unsure of how much work I should be doing and when. As a part-time student, I felt a little 'removed' from the institutional environment. I wondered, Am I doing enough? Have I read enough? Have I read the right things? Am I doing what I am supposed to be?

These kinds of question are normal for all students irrespective of their full- or part-time status, but feeling outside the institution and out of contact with the sources of information can provide answers to these worrying concerns. It may also be the case that you feel you are not getting the same kind of service as full-time counterparts or that you are not exposed to the same opportunities. Claire Maxwell was working full-time as a social worker whilst doing her PhD, and living two hours away from the university where she was enrolled was also a disadvantage. Claire describes how isolation manifests itself:

> The lack of connection with my university department meant I was very isolated. I had no one to discuss issues arising out of my research or to debate new ideas with. I felt as if I lacked the opportunity for intellectual stimulation.

Luckily, with most business conducted by email these days, you are likely to be hooked into the opportunities that the department is offering for all students. It is also an illusion that you are cutoff from a lively environment of solidarity and co-operation between colleagues. PhD study is a varied entity and people are often all over the place, doing fieldwork, teaching, working, taking time out, working at home or simply choosing to spend less time in the department. You are probably missing out on less than you think! In addition, the periodic monitoring and evaluation of your progress will enable training needs to be identified and specific areas of concern to be raised with supervisors.

Not enough hours in the day

An obvious issue, more so than for the full-time student, is that of time and juggling the many jobs that have to fit into the day. Sally Ann Halliday reflects on how the first year of her studies was fraught with clashes between work commitments and supervisory meetings:

> Over the past year it has been busy times at work and work has clashed with meetings with supervisors. 'Time', I have found, without a doubt, is the biggest hurdle to overcome. That is, making the time, then setting aside time, and then being disciplined to use it effectively.

Mothers who are involved in academia will no doubt particularly find the issue of time management a struggle. Leonard (2001: 77) makes specific references to the time issue in relation to female doctorate students, making the point that PhD study cannot just be fitted into odd hours here and there or weekends. Study needs to be organised in concentrated chunks and preferably in a space where work can be left, awaiting your return.

BOX 12.2

Remember and accept that most things will take you months to complete – not days or even weeks – when you are doing a PhD part-time. [Claire Maxwell]

A different timeframe

Doing a PhD part-time means that a different timeframe is applied to the same tasks. For instance, rather than one year for preparing the research design, literature review and methodology, this is extended to between 18 months and 24 months. Likewise with the fieldwork stage, the time for data collection is expanded, which can be a disadvantage as fieldwork often relies on momentum and immersion 'in the field'. Claire Maxwell found that the fieldwork was particularly onerous because there was no opportunity really to get involved and get the job done:

> My data collection stretched out over 15 months, as I only had a limited amount of time to pursue contacts and negotiate access. More importantly, at the data analysis and writing up stage, I often found I only had the weekends, or one day to immerse myself in my data and develop my ideas, separated by one to two weeks where my work commitments required my full attention. This lack of opportunity to immerse myself in the research process did leave me feeling like I was missing out on something – but the reality of the situation was I had to work and I actually really enjoyed that too.

Pacing yourself is something that is learnt along the way but it is a good idea to have a clear overview of what the whole project will look like on a part-time basis. Institutions all have their own regulations in relation to how long 'part-time' will take. This is generally between five and six years. Having a clear sense of the milestones you need to reach month by month can be visualised in a timetable format spelling out the jobs to be completed each year. Milestones such as upgrades, presenting at conferences, starting fieldwork, analysis and starting writing up can clearly be identified over the months.

Timetabling activities and events is important on several levels. Think about how your project will be managed over its whole lifecourse as well as revising and working to a shorter timetable in between supervisions.

The reality of juggling a job with study

Above we have outlined the obvious pitfalls of taking on two jobs simultaneously, but what are the solutions to these familiar issues? Again, we refer you to other chapters in the book, in particular Chapter 8 on Networking, Chapter 11 on Non-Traditional Routes, Chapter 9 on Missing the Deadline and Chapter 18 on Coping with Stress.

A useful framework of competencies has been offered by Rickards (1992: 44), which can be applied as a set of areas to consider if embarking on part-time study:

- Personal and life competencies (managing time, money, stress, personal relationships and domestic management).
- Work, study and academic competencies (managing work and study relationships), receptive skills (reading and listening), productive skills (writing and speaking).
- Research skills and subject competencies.

Alongside these competencies we want to emphasise some tips that have been tried and tested by our contributors.

Prioritisation

Returning to the theme of managing different jobs at the same time, a useful principle to organise your studies by is that of prioritisation. There will always be competing demands in your life whether it be children, a partner, relatives, health, finances, living arrangements, holidays, leisure, shopping, socialising – the list is endless. Each of these life elements needs to be balanced with the tasks of the PhD, which ultimately means prioritising different demands at different times. Sallyann Halliday summarises how she worked out a system of prioritisation 18 months into her studies:

To overcome the barrier of finding time to study I decided to set aside at least one day of my week to my PhD study. This is when I dedicate my whole day to doing nothing else but study. There are always other things that demand my time – shopping, sport, family and friends – but I have to be strict with myself. Even when I feel studying should be at the bottom of my 'to do' list, I have to make a conscious effort to bring it further to the top. This is not a 'breeze' – but reminding myself why I am undertaking PhD study is a great way of motivating myself to get down to it.

The personal compromises will come when you have to make decisions about what to keep in your life and what to shelve or give up for a short time. For instance, hobbies, sports, travel, socialising and additional work such as volunteering may have to be withdrawn while you get going with your study. Doing lots of things not to the best of your ability is often more frustrating than not doing them at all. Yet prioritising is difficult when lots of things are important in life and demand your attention. Claire Maxwell reflects that one of the biggest battles of managing a PhD part-time with the rest of her life was with her own feelings of guilt:

> One of the most enduring battles during my five years of doing a PhD was with myself! I constantly struggled with myself when trying to determine how much, if any, free time I should have every week. For instance, 'Did I have time to go to the gym or should I spend another hour studying?'; 'Should I agree to go for coffee with my friend, or should I stay at home and study?' Everyone who has been a student knows that feeling of guilt when you are relaxing and not studying. I carried that feeling of guilt most of the time, but when it was making me particularly miserable, I would just stop, give myself a break and do something else.

The emotional roller-coaster is often more acute for the part-time student because the job of juggling demands can become emotionally exhausting and there are times when something has to give. Recognising when you need a break from studying, or time out from juggling the madness, is as important as sticking to a tight timetable. Often taking a break from studying can mean that you are fresher and more productive when you return.

Time management

Time is a pressure for all research students. This becomes most noticeable when the writing up stage begins and it is clear that hours in front of a computer can only produce a few hundred words of progress. Writing up also means thinking time and this is where you will realise that a few odd hours here and there is simply not enough to get the job done. A concentrated period of time is needed to work on writing, editing, thinking and developing theory. Claire Maxwell offers her experience of how she negotiated extended amounts of time from her day job to concentrate on the writing stage:

I began to slowly build up my flexi-time hours until I had enough to take a whole week off in one go. I tried to ensure I had one whole week off every five or six weeks during the writing up stage to really keep the momentum going. Of course not everyone is fortunate enough to be in such a position where they are able to pretty much manage their own work schedule – but if you are – it can make a real difference. If that had not been possible, I would have considered taking some unpaid time off work during the writing up stage to keep the momentum of this phase going without too many other pressures and interruptions.

BOX 12.4   Target setting

Set yourself 'realistic' targets to achieve in your doctoral study time which take account of your personal circumstances (job, caring, family commitments). Is it realistic for you to do a few hours a day? Or is it realistic to set aside one day a week as your 'study day'? Choose whichever is most practical, then you're more likely to commit to the time slot and stick to it. [Sallyann Halliday]

Support and networking

Seeking out mechanisms of support often falls to the responsibility of the student. This can be done within the framework of the existing university or department, or other networks set up regionally and nationally can be a useful source of intellectual and emotional support. Claire Maxwell found that a specific national network that specialised in her topic was stimulating both in terms of ideas and reassurance of the PhD process:

I overcame the sense of isolation by joining a national postgraduate research support group for students studying adolescence, set up by the Trust for the Study of Adolescence. Once a term they held meetings in London, where we heard presentations about 'my research' or 'the viva', followed by small group discussions exploring different stages of the research process.

Other tips on networking and peer support in Chapter 8 are important as well as recognising that your part-time status may well enhance the need for certain coping strategies. Using your supervisor, the various programmes of training that are available for all students, as well as occasions such as seminars, workshops and postgraduate conferences, are important networking opportunities and a chance to ask questions and realise that others are in the same boat.

BOX 12.5

The average number of supervisions a part-time student can expect is about five each year. Discuss from the outset the nature of these meetings and the work expectations around them.

Key Points to Remember

▶ Part-time students often choose topics close to their employment interests.
▶ Part-time study means applying a different timeframe to the tasks, which may take months rather than weeks to complete.
▶ Prioritising studies is an important organising principle.
▶ Chunks of time are essential not odd hours here and there.
▶ Having a clear timetable and set of milestones will make the years seem more structured.
▶ Networking is even more important to prevent negative isolation as a part-time student.

SUGGESTED READING

De Fazio, T. (2002) *Studying Part Time Without Stress*. London: Allen & Unwin.
Gatrell, C. (2006) *Managing Part-Time Study*. Maidenhead: Open University Press.
Pritchard, L. with Roberts, L. (2006) *The Mature Student's Guide to Higher Education*. Maidenhead: Open University Press.
Rose, J. (2001) *The Mature Student's Guide to Writing* Basingstoke: Palgrave.

Chapter 13

Combining Teaching and Doctoral Studies

What this Chapter Includes:

▶ How teaching undergraduates fits into doing a PhD
▶ The clear benefits of teaching to your research and career
▶ How to prevent teaching interfering with your PhD
▶ Dealing with 'bad teaching days'
▶ Effective corner-cutting that doesn't reduce quality
▶ Suggestions for when teaching is not available

The unsaid assumption

Over the past decade, teaching undergraduates while conducting a doctorate has become a familiar experience. There is a 'long established tradition of casual teaching by doctoral students' (Phillips and Pugh, 2005: 91), that means teaching is often an expectation of departments. Now that doctorates are financially supported through teaching bursaries or scholarships that encourage departments to provide teaching experience as part of the award, it is rare for postgraduates not to be offered teaching. It is not only the change in the overall philosophy of what a doctorate is that has driven this change. With more academics holding 'buy-outs' from normal duties and increasing undergraduate numbers, the demand for teaching staff is considerable and many programmes, especially in research-led universities, could not run without this contingent of casual labour that turns up every September (Holt, 1999).

Until recently, rarely has the combination of teaching and doing a PhD been reflected upon as traditionally there has been an assumption that academics are natural teachers. From our own experience of sitting in lectures we know this is far from the truth! There has been a neglect of *how* the teaching is done because it is assumed that academics have the expertise in the subject that will give them the skills necessary to teach. From other quarters there have been concerns raised about ensuring that postgraduates who are employed in Higher Education get a fair deal. Unions have got together to write the Employed Postgraduates' Charter (2003), which calls for some of the following rights:

- Non-discriminatory appointment procedures.
- Written statement of terms and conditions.
- Belonging to a trade union of choice.
- Pay for all responsibilities and work undertaken.
- Full departmental and institutional integration.

What has also been sidelined is the special relationships between postgraduates teaching undergraduates, which is different from when full-time members of the academic teaching staff are conversing with students. Teaching when you are a post-graduate brings with it a set of dynamics that are complex. If postgraduates have only recently finished their undergraduate studies there are issues of role conflict as well as concerns that the teacher is virtually the same age as the students. Whatever age you start teaching it can be daunting, and this is not always appreciated. At the minimum, institutions should offer basic training in teaching methods and assessment for instance, as well as regular feedback and support sessions. We are aware that this is not generally the case. From a study of postgraduate teachers at the University of Otago, New Zealand, the vast majority of interviewees (71%) reported no formal training (Harland and Plangger, 2004: 76). This is despite evidence from 22 universities in the UK that training university teachers increased the extent to which the teacher adopts a student focus teaching style, improving the outcomes for the students (Gibbs and Coffey, 2004).

There have been concerns raised by the Higher Education Academy and the government about the need to ensure that postgraduates who are teaching are fully trained. The Government White Paper *The Future of Higher Education* stated that all new teaching staff should receive accredited training by 2006 (Department for Education and Skills, 2003: 46). To support this aim, a set of professional standards was introduced in 2006 (The UK Professional Standards Framework for Supporting Teaching and Learning in Higher Education), which emphasises a high quality student learning experience and the professional development of staff engaged in teaching. To achieve this at the University of Leeds, postgraduate students who teach in their second year are offered a course called the 'Modules in Learning and Teaching in Higher Education for Postgraduates and other Part Time Teachers' (NDTHLE), which consists of workshops, peer observation, assessed work and mentoring.

BOX 13.1 The whole teaching experience can be considered in four ways:

- The training
- Preparation
- The delivery
- Career development

What is teaching?

There are a plethora of different teaching tasks that postgraduates are asked to undertake. This can range from laboratory demonstrations, one-to-one supervision of dissertations and project work, assisting in IT or study skills workshops, or even giving a lecture. Most often, students are needed to conduct seminar or tutorial work. Modules normally operate with a one hour lecture each week given by the module convenor (usually a full-time academic) and then a one-hour tutorial that accompanies the topic. The postgraduate-teacher organises and delivers the tutorial aimed at dissecting the topic to get students to think more critically about the issue. John Roberts explains what this actually entails:

> In the social sciences and humanities you will probably be asked to teach first year seminars. Seminars are structured around a set of key readings. Obviously you must complete this reading. From this reading you should be able to gain a list of questions to ask the students during the seminar. Or from the reading you might think of a number of examples from everyday life that will illustrate points from the main reading.

Increasingly, first year teaching is returning to some basic study skills such as essay writing, presentation skills, referencing and bibliographies (students get this wrong no matter how many times they are told!). You may be required to teach some of these formally but if not you can always integrate them into your tutorials.

Whether you are teaching a subject on which you consider yourself a bit of an expert, or whether it is all new material, getting some guidance and direction before you start is essential. This should be formalised, although John Roberts reflects how sometimes postgraduate teaching staff are overlooked:

> When I started teaching as a postgraduate student at universities no full-time academic member of staff ever took me to one side to tell me how to teach or how to mark. Somehow you are supposed to miraculously know how to do both. Be prepared for this and realise that you are doing the department a favour as much as they are doing you a favour.

It is important to be clear from the start what your role is and where the boundaries are drawn. Check what your contract states and if you are not happy with the workload or expected duties then see if this can be negotiated. Morss and Murray (2005: 3) outline what is *not* the responsibility of the teaching assistant:

- To read every paper on the topic.
- To design the curriculum.
- To write or re-write the syllabus.
- To take responsibility for the students.
- To design assessments.

BOX 13.2   Training to teach is essential

If training is not offered then demand it! If it is offered make sure you are paid for under-taking it.

Whether you are on a teaching bursary or taking on casual teaching duties, Phillips and Pugh (2005: 92) suggest good practice is to obtain a letter of appointment which specifies the tasks and hourly rates. Teaching bursaries may hold special 'Terms and Conditions' from the university which are different for those for taking on casual teaching. These differ widely between universities and departments so check what they are before you sign up. JK Tina Basi, who taught throughout her four years as a PhD student, suggests all postgraduate teachers clarify their role by asking some of these questions:

Will you have flexibility over what to teach? What will the marking consist of? Will you need to set open door hours or attend lectures? How much administrative work is required? Will you need to take staff training courses? How often, if at all, will you meet the module convenor or other Teaching Assistants? It is important that you get the answers to your questions earlier rather than later.

Also, make sure you are aware of the number of hours you will be expected to teach. The National Postgraduate Committee guidelines suggests no more than six hours per week per semester. The research councils suggest very similar teaching loads.

So, what's in it for me?

Let's be honest, one of the main motivating factors for teaching is the cash (this may transfer into fees or a scholarship)! Casual staff in universities are paid decent money, and marking essays and exams is usually paid per script. But there are also positive reasons for teaching that spread beyond a solution for the cash-flow problem. There are other academic-related benefits that should convince you that taking on a teaching load is worth it. Yousaf Ibrahim experienced teaching as an essential part of the PhD process:

> Right from the outset teaching has been a major advantage for me during the PhD process in three ways: access to resources and funding; confidence building, especially when deciding on your PhD topic; and acquiring knowledge through teaching, which informed my research and by undertaking research I developed my own specialism in teaching – in effect a virtuous cycle.

There are some specific advantages to teaching undergraduates that can assist you in your theoretical development for the thesis. In addition, you can make clear links between your own research and teaching. These points will be explored below.

Reading the classics

Teela Sanders, who has responsibility for managing teaching assistants, notes how many students reflect time after time that even though it was sometimes a bind, teaching actually took them back to the reading they should have done at the beginning of the doctorate. If we have been studying a discipline for several years before we even come to the doctorate, we can have quite a jaded relationship with the 'founding fathers' of the discipline. However, whether we like it or not these texts are integral to understanding the wider context of your study area and revisiting them in order to teach elementary theories and concepts can be a blessing in disguise. JK Tina Basi describes how returning to core textbooks and original manuscripts that could be considered a chore was turned into a positive contribution to the PhD:

> Teaching first year students in what amounts to the basics of your discipline is not only a good refresher and reminder of how your work can contribute overall to the academy, but the experience feeds into your own research in unexpected and exciting ways. Students bring a fresh approach to theories that might appear stale and insufficient in your own research and will often ask questions that push you to think laterally around your own subject area.

Use the undergraduate reading lists to start the PhD literature review. Getting back to the classics can be a real eye opener and lead your thinking in new directions.

Enhancing the research

The skills that can be developed through teaching (both those acquired from training and those natural skills that are developed) are transferable to many aspects of the PhD process. For instance, talking confidently to a group of people is a necessary part of presenting a paper at a conference or conducting fieldwork. Also, learning how to answer questions that are thrown at you and being able to 'think on your feet' is another good skill to learn in preparation for presentations and the viva. Robertson and Bond (2001) make the point that research informs teaching while at the same time teaching becomes a channel for knowledge transfer. Yousaf Ibrahim found clear crossovers between his empirical data collection and teaching:

As soon as I started to carry out my research I found clear links between this and the subjects I was teaching. Having carried out fieldwork I was able to share real empirical experience with students on a whole range of issues associated with strategy, design and implementation. This gave added value to my teaching. It also worked the other way round, my teaching informed my research objectives and questions.

Other skills you develop whilst teaching undergraduates can be more directly relevant to gathering data and conducting fieldwork. Marta Bolognani, who was conducting an ethnographic anthropological study, makes this clear:

Group work in the tutorials helped me to develop skills that I implemented when running focus groups for my fieldwork. One of the most rewarding experiences I went through was negotiating to run focus groups in a secondary school. By taking advantage of my experience in teaching I was able to strike a deal with the teachers: I would run one-hour revision for the class and they would take part in a one-hour focus group. There I implemented group work strategies that I had developed through my teaching experience.

Access to resources

When you register for a doctorate you have a specific student contract with the university, whereas when you take on a teaching contract (even if casual) you become a member of staff. Although this does not mean you have full entitlements like other full-time staff, it certainly can provide a welcome route to resources that are otherwise a financial burden for a student. Yousaf Ibrahim describes how taking on a dual role in the department has hidden benefits:

> As a member of staff I had access to many resources. I had, at least some of the time, office space, a desk, telephone, Internet and e-mail access. I had access to library books, journal articles with a longer loan period and a generous photocopying allowance. Having regular contact with colleagues who had been through the PhD process, especially the viva, was an important communication line to pass on important advice.

Career development

If you have dreams of becoming a fully fledged member of the academy after your doctorate, then you cannot escape teaching. Nor should you want to as teaching, research and writing are intricately linked. Such a relationship allegedly has Harvard professors fighting to get onto the first year teaching timetable. The point is, teaching is necessary for your CV and if you can teach at least first years (with experience you could progress to other levels), then you have secured a decent reference from a senior member of staff who can testify your teaching proficiency. Indeed, by the time you apply for jobs you may well have some snazzy module outlines sitting on your PC ready to be rolled out in the next academic year. However, in the mass education system that is Higher Education, be prepared to be accountable. Your teaching is evaluated by the following methods:

- Student evaluation questionnaires.
- Peer observation and feedback from mentor.
- Marking is 'second' marked by another member of staff.

In the age where undergraduates are paying fees to be taught, the quality of teaching and accountability of those who provide it will only increase. However, this is all about developing the skill of 'knowledge transfer'. It is useful to see teaching as part of the postgraduate experience as you are both a developing 'expert' yet remain a 'learner' (Harland and Plangger, 2004: 78). Drawing on experiences of postgraduate teachers, Harland and Plangger (2004: 81) describe a range of identities experienced during the role as individuals move between 'students, learners, teachers, researchers or academics', likening the experience to one of being a chameleon.

BOX 13.5

Teaching experience is essential for your CV if you want to apply for an academic post.

And the catch is?

With all opportunities there are drawbacks that could make the progression of your PhD frustrating. Inevitably while you are spending time on preparing and delivering teaching you are not reading that article or writing that next chapter. This section will explore how teaching can interfere with the PhD and provides tips to steer you away from this familiar concern.

Interference with the PhD

Reflecting on several years of teaching whilst completing the PhD, John Roberts explains how hours designated to teaching can leak into days and suddenly you have lost considerable PhD time:

> Just teaching one seminar at, say, midday, can lead to a substantial amount of time away from PhD research. First there is the build up to teaching the seminar – making sure you have your notes on the subject, the questions you want to ask, and so on. Second, there is the actual teaching of the seminar. And finally the time afterwards in which you want to wind down after teaching by taking an extended lunch break!

Above we see some very realistic concerns outlined where teaching can end up being the sole focus of the week, relegating the PhD to evenings and weekends. If this happens the balance needs to be turned around, so that while you are still engaged in teaching, your doctorate is at the forefront of your energies. It's a difficult juggling act. However, the answers lie mainly with time management (there are always in-house courses on this for postgraduates, so if you think this is an issue – don't be shy). JK Tina Basi advises against getting over-enthusiastic about planning and preparation:

> Your first concern in balancing teaching and doctoral studies will be in time management. It is very easy to get excited and energetic about creating and designing activities that will stimulate students. It is very important that teaching doesn't begin to become more of a focus than your own research so it's best to set aside some time during the week for preparation and administration and do your best not to go over that time.

BOX 13.6

To minimise the amount of time spent teaching, pack all of your teaching into one day so that you can devote as many full and clear days as possible to your PhD research.

A bad teaching day

You will almost certainly experience a 'bad teaching day', when no one turns up, or if they do they look at you as if you are an alien, or you end up speaking till you are hoarse because your students are doing a great impression of a silent movie! It is all just part of the ebb and flow of the teaching experience. If you have followed advice you will have some tricks up your sleeve to prevent the deadly silence, but even to the most experienced, sometimes teaching is difficult and stressful. JK Tina Basi shares some of her more stressful moments, suggesting this is far from unusual:

> It is totally normal to have a bad teaching session when students have not done the reading and do not feel like speaking, or when everyone feels like speaking and the situation feels out of control. It is important to remember that it is not a reflection of how well you know the material or how good you are at teaching. Just remember that everyone has bad days, including students. Don't be surprised if you need a shoulder to cry on on more than one occasion.

Teaching is a responsible job and can sometimes be overwhelming – so when you feel like drowning your sorrows or indulging in self-pity, make sure you speak to your peers as they will all have had the same experience. Just remember the satisfaction should outweigh the stressful, emotional aspect of teaching, you may not think so immediately, but in time it will prove to have been worth it.

BOX 13.7

To prevent deathly silence in tutorials, always have some pre-planned exercises for the class. This could be study skills or newspaper-based work.

Effective corner-cutting strategies

Our contributors, three of whom were still in the throes of teaching whilst doing their doctorates when they wrote these pieces, can offer some teaching tips for those who are about to get involved with juggling the two jobs of teaching and researching.

Beware Not to Over-Prepare

When faced with a huge reading list, a room full of eager undergraduates, or a theorist to explain whom you have never heard of, there is a great tendency to spend several days reading all you can in order to feel you can get through a 45-minute seminar. Hold your horses! Spending too much time preparing makes this whole endeavour financially inefficient and interferes with the flow of your PhD. Learning how to prepare enough in the minimum amount of time is the primary skill you need to perfect. John Roberts and Yousaf Ibrahim offer some advice on how to prepare efficiently and still feel confident about the quality of your teaching:

> The main point to remember in order to save you too much work is try to think of how you can prepare well for the seminar without having to do too much background reading. This is all the more important once you realise that many seminar topics that you will have to teach will be areas that you may not be too familiar with. [John Roberts]
>
> I made sure I ring-fenced and protected my time. The days for preparation of teaching, associated administration and research should be kept separate. Draw up a timetable and commit so many hours to teaching preparation. Remember though too much research and no social contact with neither students nor colleagues can be very isolating, and too much teaching and not enough research on your PhD can cause panic and anxiety in the sense that you feel you are not getting on with your own work. [Yousaf Ibrahim]

Your preparation not only means learning the topic so you feel confident enough to summarise what was in the lecture and spark debate. You need to think about strategies to get the students talking, as you are the facilitator of their learning. John Roberts offers some simple, but effective strategies:

One good strategy to achieve this is to place the emphasis upon the students. For example, I sometimes used to get students into groups, give them some questions for discussion about a particular reading, and then have a wider discussion at the end.

Repetition is a useful tool to cut down on preparation time. JK Tina Basi summarises how the main goal of the seminars is for the students to do the work, while you act as a mindful shepherd(ess) guiding them through the pastures:

A top tip in combining teaching and doctoral studies is to prepare one seminar or tutorial and repeat it for all of your groups. Try not to do all the work and get your students involved by having them sign up to do presentations – it ensures their presence and participation in class. Above all remember that you are not there to provide them with a lecture or do their reading for them – you are there to stimulate and manage a group discussion. They need to meet you half way!

BOX 13.8

Be prepared to say 'NO' to extra work that you deem unfair or outside your agreed contract.

Marking – get it out of the way

Marking can sometimes be more stressful than actually taking the seminars as you are making a judgement on someone's piece of work which could affect their final degree classification. Remember that you have to be accountable, which is why there are guidelines for all assessors and an in-house and external marking process to make sure there are no anomalies. Again, get guidance from the module convenor and peers as to the best strategy to mark accurately and effectively. Often marking has to fit to tight deadlines, so putting it off should not be an option. John Roberts explains the process in more depth:

Marking coursework can take a few days, especially when marking batches of first year essays, as these comprise the largest number of students in a degree scheme. Even though marking may seem a somewhat laborious task it is best to get them marked and returned as soon as possible. Each department should have its own guidelines about what constitutes a First, a 2.1, 2.2, and so on. Work from these guidelines because students would most likely have read them as well and so will write essays accordingly.

Be careful not to get roped into looking at drafts of work, or spending so much time with students that you have co-written the essay. Students can sometimes be persistent, so have clear boundaries in terms of how much time you will spend advising individual students.

What if teaching is not available?

Sometimes teaching may not be available to you, but you may feel that you want this experience for career development reasons. Here are a few options:

If you can't do any teaching in your Department and you are interested in experiencing teaching young people, see if the local council runs mentoring schemes or check on the ESRC website whether they would support you as a 'Researcher in Residence' in a secondary school or 6th form college.
[Marta Bolognani]

The Open University are always looking for Associate Lecturers to run their distance learning courses. This teaching is slightly different from the conventional university style as it involves marking essays, running a handful of tutorials throughout the course and assisting students, normally via the telephone or email. It is worth putting in an application a year before you want to teach just so you are on the books. (See www.openuniversity.ac.uk)
[Teela Sanders]

▶ Check opportunities for teaching before you register, or if you are funded through a teaching bursary then check the terms and conditions. Always clarify the teaching role whatever your status.

▶ Think beyond the payslip. There are real benefits to teaching in terms of helping to develop your research, thesis and thinking.

▶ Make links between your own research experience and teaching, keeping it fresh and offering real examples to undergraduates.

▶ If you want to apply for an academic post, then teaching is essential on your CV.

▶ Teaching is a skill and you need training and support.

▶ Don't let teaching take over your week or your PhD. Be strict with timetabling and ring-fence your preparation time.

▶ Enjoy your contact with students – passing on knowledge is a privilege and fun. After all, everyone remembers a good teacher.

SUGGESTED READING

Harland, T. and Plangger, G. (2004) 'The postgraduate chameleon', *Active Learning in Higher Education,* 5 (1): 73–86.

Morss, K. and Murray, R. (2005) *Teaching at University: A Guide for Postgraduates and Researchers.* London: Sage.

Chapter 14

Reconciling the Research Role with the Personal

What this Chapter Includes:

▶ Doctoral research and the 'personal'
▶ Biography, lived experiences and the personal as research
▶ Emotions and doing research
▶ Emotions in the field
▶ Emotional responses throughout the research process
▶ Being aware of and managing your emotions

Doctoral research and the 'personal'

This chapter explores the doctoral process as an emotional and personal experience. We seek to take a more holistic view of research students who make an emotional and personal investment in their research project. We look at the converging relationships between your research and the rest of your life as well as some aspects of tension, stress and conflict. Many advice and guidance books recognise that doctoral research not only involves personal motivations and investments but also requires managing your approach to your study in a proactive way and in ways that support your other personal aspirations, well-being and commitments. Hence, doctoral study guides discuss strategies for time management, generating a research–home balance and being aware of your personal well-being beyond your research aspirations (see Wilkinson, 2005; Wisker, 2001). Many have remarked that succeeding in completing your PhD will inevitably involve a journey of 'peaks and troughs', 'highs and lows' as well as sacrifice, discipline, persistence, hard work and effort on your part (Phillips and Pugh, 2005).

Viewing the research student as an emotional being immersed in wider social relationships is rarely apparent in research method discussions. Guidelines for research conduct and methods can be aimed at a rather one-dimensional 'researcher' – devoid of multiple life roles, experiences and priorities. This can be due to adherence to a theoretical or 'scientific' approach that seeks to establish a purely rational and 'objective' stance towards knowledge production, but it is also because personal emotions and our lives outside of the 'research role' are viewed as a private and individual matter – something for discussion between peers, family members or friends rather than for public inquiry or institutional intervention. While we are not seeking to provide a stance on such issues, here we are concerned to give space and recognition to the connections between our wider selves (as more than analytical beings or full-time researchers), lives and relationships for two reasons. First, because it is across these multiple spheres that we live, and events, relationships and routines in everyday life shape the nitty-gritty of everyday research practice. Secondly, because for research students, undertaking an apprenticeship, it is perhaps even more vital and pertinent to be aware of their emotional inner world and seek to manage this interface in ways that aid personal development and research progress. Because of the significance of the tensions and transgressions between our 'personal lives' and the research endeavour, we have made similar points in other chapters in this book, especially in this present section and in Part IV, which follows, including discussions on doing a PhD as part of a career change, undertaking a PhD part-time and juggling doctoral research with caring commitments.

There are five aspects of this more embedded, personalised and holistic view of the doctorate process and student. First, as we discussed in Chapter 1, undertaking a PhD arises out of personal motivations and investments whether these involve aspirations for an ongoing academic career or a more personal intellectual curiosity. Secondly, you will be immersed in and have to engage with the personal motivations and micro-level 'emotions' of your institutional and disciplinary relationships. Thirdly, research demands you invest yourself in the process. It is an intensely personal endeavour as a researcher is not just an analytical person, but has their own hopes and fears. Much of what you do as a researcher involves presenting oneself in particular ways and proactively shaping the research. Research involves engagement at an intellectual level as well as in an emotional and personal capacity. You may expect yourself to give a high level of commitment and others, such as your supervisors, will certainly communicate such expectations to you also. Such absorption can be very consuming and ultimately rewarding in the event of completing your research and gaining the doctorate. However, even if we so desired, most of us do not live in a world where we can isolate ourselves for the duration of our study! Not only will the everyday experience of doing a PhD be a personally and emotionally engaging experience, your research pre-occupations and roles are likely to have an impact on those you are close to and other spheres of your life – as well as these spheres and others having an impact on you as a researcher.

Fourthly, undertaking doctoral research is becoming more about ongoing personal development and career progression. Again the specific types of skills and orientations you wish to develop will be highly individualistic as you will be building on your prior capacities and aiming to achieve new skills suitable to your future plans. Lastly, these aspects of the research process can actually form the central part of your analytical inquiries – as is the case within autobiographical or reflexively driven research approaches.

Biography, lived experiences and the personal as research

These five aspects demonstrating the embedded and personal nature of the doctoral experience and endeavour were illuminated by our case study contributors. Many demonstrated how their research interests had emerged from their own experiences as an ongoing part of their 'life projects'. Our previous life experiences and attitudes can often stimulate our interest in specific research areas. Within the social sciences it is common for our personal experiences to motivate us towards looking at particular areas as substantive research issues. This can provide much motivation but will also mean that your connections to the subject are complex and multifaceted. Taking a critical stance you will need to think through your prior knowledge, assumptions, values and feelings on the subject. For example, Sonali Shah felt her PhD topic on disabled women 'high flyers' expressed her own political and social concerns and beliefs as well as her own aspirations towards an academic career. Her intellectual endeavours were a deeply personal matter:

> The experiences of myself, of friends and of other disabled people working against disabling barriers within a mainstream society motivated me to do research in this area. I was eager to develop work that reflected my personal belief that every person has the right to their freedom to make personal choices, in accordance with their personal credentials, and not to be stereotyped in any way. The PhD experience was not only the key to the start of a successful career in academia, it was key for a happy and successful life.

Your research questions and activities may not arise directly from your own personal experiences – and they may then further inform your life interests and outlook. Not only will your research activities have an impact on you, the demands of your research will need to be balanced against other life commitments. Claire Maxwell, for example, discusses her need to study her PhD part-time while also developing her career as a social worker:

> Studying part-time was the only option for me as I wanted to work as a social worker. Furthermore, I needed to earn money to cover my living expenses no matter what. At this point in time, my commitment lay in developing a career as a social worker, with the PhD almost occupying the space of a pastime.

> **BOX 14.1   What kind of life project would PhD research be for you?**
>
> Being aware of what investments you are willing and able to make into your doctoral research may help reveal your expectations, competing commitments and motivations. Ask yourself:
>
> - What are your reasons for doing a PhD?
> - How you expect your PhD research to impact on the rest of your life?
> - What is the right kind of balance between doing the PhD and the rest of your life that you wish to achieve?

Some methodological approaches demand more of a critical reflexivity among researchers, where you reflect on and analyse your role in shaping and framing your research. For example, you could be undertaking research with a concern to explicitly analyse the role of the researcher within the research process, such as the role of the researcher's values and assumptions about human behaviour or social relations that emerge from the researcher's own biographical experiences. Reflecting on your particular input into the research process will be important here. The researcher extends the analysis towards their own inner worlds using techniques to note down, capture and think through emotions and identifications with your research area (see Ribbens and Edwards, 1998; Letherby, 2003).

> **BOX 14.2   Think about the relationship between your wider life experiences and your research activities/topic**
>
> These questions may help:
>
> - Are there some overlaps and what are the implications of these?
> - What prior knowledge and experience do you have in relation to your research topic?
> - Will you analyse your experiences and viewpoints as part of your research methodology? Why would this be worthwhile or necessary?

There could be several points of tension as well as convergence between your roles as a researcher, research student and the rest of your life. Tensions between your PhD and the rest of your life can be of a practical, emotional, ethical or intellectual nature. It may be helpful for you to consider how your commitment to your research project will be balanced against your other commitments. On the other side of the coin, what you bring to your studies, and your prior values, beliefs and orientations in undertaking research will also play a part in determining your PhD experience. In moving your research forward and balancing your multiple commitments, there is much room for conflict but also personal transformation and development.

Claire Maxwell decided to change her PhD topic because her area was personally challenging and her interests in her subject changed towards a new area:

> As I began specialising in the study of violence against women I suspected that I would 'end up' working for an organisation that campaigned in this field and wondered whether, despite my commitment to this area, this might potentially limit my future career options. Also, people's anxiety and inability to talk about (sexual) violence as well as my time at the Rape Crisis and Sexual Abuse Centre made me realise that when working in this field, the political is personal and it becomes part of who you are and how people see you. Emotionally I was not sure whether I had the energy or wanted to wear my feminist principles on my sleeve at all times, which I felt I would have to if I worked in this field. Further, after having worked with young people as a social worker for over a year, I had become more and more interested in the world of youth.

On the other hand, Sonali Shah notes that she developed many personal skills while undertaking PhD research, including 'endurance, persistence and standing up for [her] own rights to institutional support as a disabled student': 'The five years I spent working on my PhD has proved to be a crucial period of personal development for me. It has taken me into new avenues of competence, and exposed me to great inspirations.' Doing a doctorate is not a cut and dry analytical or intellectual endeavour. You will learn new things about yourself and your capacities (or even limits!). It is a personal journey as much as an intellectual one.

Emotions and doing research

In examining the role played by our emotional inner worlds in the research process, we will now look at three features – emotions in the field, emotional investments and emotional responses. The subsequent section then explores possibilities for managing and coping with these emotional sides of the research process.

Emotions in the field
Embarking on fieldwork and engaging in relationships with others outside of the world of research or university life can bring about many issues and circumstances that simply cannot be planned or prepared for. Fieldwork relationships, perhaps more

pronounced in qualitative research approaches, involve meeting real people and engaging with them. You will be faced with your own emotional responses as well as the emotional needs and responses of others. The contributors to this book described both negative and positive emotional reactions and situations emerging from their fieldwork experiences. As previously discussed, Ruth Bartlett felt empathy with the welfare and service needs of her interviewees, who were older people with dementia. She felt torn between her emotional and health professional reactions to her clients' stories of their care needs and experiences, while also recognising the limitations of her capacities to help within her researcher role. Further, Ruth felt concerned about the emotional implications of her research methods, using in-depth interviews, on the research participants, who may rarely be asked such personally revealing questions for research purposes. Qualitative interviewing is hence an intensely demanding process for researcher and interviewee. As we reviewed in Chapters 2 and 4, it is important to think through the likely emotional and personal impact of your research methods on your participants and check out possible avenues for providing information on professional support services if difficult memories or emotions arise for the interviewee or yourself.

Other contributors described their attachment to the fieldwork experience and interactions with real life experiences. Sonali Shah felt inspired and in awe of her research participants: 'Although the PhD work was demanding, and challenging, often leaving me exhausted, frustrated and wanting to quit, I was greatly inspired by the disabled high-flyers who participated in my study.' Below and elsewhere in this volume (especially in Part IV) we consider the significance of seeking support for dealing with and recognising the legitimacy of such emotional experiences. Undertaking fieldwork can be a time when a researcher feels quite alone, needing to think for themselves and on their feet, away from their supervisor or peers. Rebecca Mallett warns against dismissing worries, as thinking these through and sharing them may help you to progress and learn:

> Like all postgraduates 'in the field', I was left to my own devices but my devices were not capable of coping. I felt under immense pressure not to admit this and not to ask for advice and support. A mistake I would not encourage anyone else to make.

Emotional responses throughout the research process

We found that several of our contributors referred to a wide range of emotions such as anxiety, fear, excitement, panic, shame and pride – several of which have been raised in earlier chapters. For example, common sources of anxiety could be:

- Presenting your ideas to supervisors, higher status academics or large audiences.
- Contemplating a change in method or topic.

- Negotiating the terms of fieldwork with outside individuals or organisations.
- Networking.
- Monitoring progress.
- Undertaking a task for the first time.
- Seeking advice and supervision.

Starting out as a doctoral research student can particularly be a time of personal transition, involving uncertainty and shaky self-confidence. It is an academic apprenticeship, and it is not surprising to feel a lack of confidence at the beginning stages of a learning process. Harriet Churchill felt she was not a traditional PhD student, having returned to Higher Education after several years looking after her young daughter full-time:

> I experienced the first year of doctoral research as a time of much self-doubt and uncertainty. Re-reading my personal journal at this time, there are many references to uncertainty about my own competence as a researcher/academic. I felt unsure if I would be able to generate an adequate study against the benchmark of 'originality' and very uncertain about what my focus would be. These perceptions were extremely anxiety-provoking. I perceived others to be much more competent than myself. My emotions led me to feel quite nervous about seeing supervisors.

The importance of this example is the way that emotions played a powerful role in how Harriet proceeded in her research and relationship with supervisors. Further, her inner world tended to involve perceptions of inadequacy that led to her feeling vulnerable and isolated. In this example, anxiety can become 'disabling and contribute to a self-fulfilling cycle of victim status' (Morley, 1999). An alternative view (albeit a very rational one in the face of powerful emotions and self-perceptions) of these difficulties could be to contemplate that such uncertainty, vulnerability and anxiety is very common in the initial stages of the research process. Rather than a sign of personal adequacy, starting out as a doctoral student may involve common experiences of anxiety over competence and progression. Acknowledging the areas and activities where you feel less competent can be an empowering process that can lead to the identification of research training needs. Uncertainty and self-doubt could lead to constructively reviewing one's need for development, one's task at hand and seeking support through training, practice, mentoring or gaining resources (Morley, 1999). Thinking about activities that trigger feelings of self-doubt and anxiety as potential areas for development can help you regain some control over your emotional reactions.

Dealing with the unexpected and working out appropriate ways to alter your research plans when the need arises can also be a common source of discomfort. Many doctoral students are just as vulnerable to the fears of failure and worries about progress that the general population may have in relation to their goals. The early stages of designing your research can particularly be hampered by a fear of developing a 'good and original proposal' as we saw in Chapter 2. Having to change your plans is likely to illustrate a close engagement with your progress, rather than failure. Changes can demonstrate flexibility and adaptation as you respond to dilemmas and constraints. Moving forward with a sense of uncertainty can be uncomfortable but adapting your plans in ways that enhance your chances of success and contribution can be viewed in quite positive ways.

Another common experience, especially in the latter part of doctoral studies, is feeling study fatigue. As an intellectual exercise and the largest thesis you are likely to submit for an examination, your PhD will inevitably be draining particularly in times of meeting deadlines or progressing towards completion. It is common for supervisors to demand students spend long hours on their studies at this point. Even if this is practical, you will feel drained and will need to think through how to sustain your energy and motivation.

Managing your emotions

The literature on personal well-being strategies for doctoral students discusses strategies for getting by and getting through the 'hard times' as well as attempting to achieve 'the right balance' between research and the rest of your life/your personal well-being (Howard et al., 2002; Wisker, 2004). Many of our contributors discussed several possible ways to overcome challenging times. A common issue was regret at 'keeping it all bottled up' which sustained a sense of isolation but also made students vulnerable to much internal anxiety, draining their energy and blocking progress. Others refer to the value of taking a break and talking things through with peers and friends. Box 14.3 begins to explore some valued options for generating awareness and overcoming problems. The following chapters in Part IV now turn to focus on the central importance of seeking appropriate and useful support.

Box 14.3   Emotional awareness and management

Strategies for gaining emotional awareness and enhancing your capacities to manage emotional reactions within the field and the research process could include:

- Regular reflection on your research activities and responses within discussions with your supervisor, your peers or in a written format in a research diary or log.
- Assessing your likes and dislikes, fears and hopes within the research process and as a critical component of research planning and design. This assessment could lead you to identify anxiety-provoking situations for you and possible ways of developing/ preparing your skills and approach.

(Continued)

- Asking others for advice and real-life examples of how they experience and respond to emotional aspects of the research process.
- Be prepared for your research to impact on yourself and your life in a multiplicity of ways.
- Be honest about your limitations and learn to say 'No' if necessary!
- Be sensitive and informed about the political and ethical nature of research.
- Try not to let your research activities damage your health, well-being or personal relationships!
- Recognise when you need support and advice and be determined to seek out the right support for you.

Key Points to Remember

▶ Doctoral research involves a personal experience that can include competing commitments as well as wider life transformations.

▶ You may have several prior assumptions and viewpoints on your research topic due to your previous life experiences.

▶ You may consider a research methodology that seeks to analyse your personal experiences and responses to your research activities.

▶ Thinking about how your doctoral studies relate to the rest of your life may help you to manage the process and plan your time.

▶ Thinking through the impact your studies have on your life may help you to recognise the connections between your doctoral research and your personal life.

SUGGESTED READING

Cryer, P. (2000) *The Research Student's Guide to Success*, 2nd edn. Buckingham: Open University Press.

Etherington, K. (2004) *Becoming a Reflexive Researcher: Using Ourselves in Research*. London: Jessica Kingsley.

Hockey, J. (1994) 'New territories: problems of adjusting to the first year of a social science PhD', *Studies in Higher Education*, 19(2): 177–190.

Marshall, S. and Green, N. (2004) *Your PhD Companion*. Oxford: How To Books.

Murray, R. (2002) *How to Write a Thesis*. Maidenhead: Open University Press.

Part IV
Relationships of Support

This final section focuses on the emotional journey of the PhD process by recognising the need for support and indicating some useful strategies for finding and nurturing those relationships. This aspect of the PhD and the place of the doctorate in your life demands particular attention, we believe, because it is often one of the taboo subjects that gets overlooked and missed off the institutional agenda. We have dedicated four chapters to uncovering the complexities of relationships of support and the obligations of institutions to support students, and we also make suggestions as to where and how this support can be accessed.

To begin, Chapter 15 returns to the relationship PhD students have with their supervisor. To be read in conjunction with Chapter 3 'Choosing and Changing Your Supervisor', Chapter 15 irons out exactly what you should expect from your supervisor, your own obligations to work with the relationship and how to use your supervisions effectively. Exploring different types and styles of supervision will give students insight into the nuances of the relationship, including a benchmark from which to measure their supervisory arrangements. Using examples from our contributors, we explore troubleshooting tips and how to manage the somewhat complex relationship with your supervisor.

Chapter 16 takes a more objective view of the wider research environment that PhD students work within. Here we examine the problems with the academic institution that can be disabling for some students, reducing opportunities for a fair and discrimination-free experience. We particularly look at the issues around institution practices, equal opportunities and how to find out your rights as a student. Looking specifically at ways in which students can be exploited in the academic institution, we highlight methods of making sure you are given the resources, time and expertise that is part of the university's contract with you.

Chapter 17 draws on some of the issues highlighted in the previous chapter by examining the increasing tendency for postgraduate students to be heavily involved in caring commitments and the obligations that come with managing and running a household. Drawing heavily on examples from men and women who have been PhD students whilst also caring for members of their immediate and extended families, the concerns of managing multiple responsibilities are addressed through a realistic perspective. We examine how doing a PhD can often be incompatible with other life commitments and roles, and how, although perhaps these problems cannot be resolved, working solutions can be found. These challenges, burdens and commitments are explored in the context of managing the academic workload and the three-year deadline.

The chapter that closes the book examines how students who take on the PhD can experience stress due to a combination of work and personal issues. Stress is examined as an occupational hazard of this job, and we hope the chapter offers comfort to those who doubt their abilities or feel that the problems are insurmountable. We identify several avenues of support, including specialist counselling services, that are available free of charge through most universities.

Chapter 15

What to Expect from Your Supervisor

What this Chapter Includes:

▶ Outline of what your supervisor should be doing
▶ What to expect in terms of support and feedback
▶ Your work expectations
▶ Your responsibility in the relationship
▶ How to use your supervisions effectively
▶ Managing your supervisor]

The basics

Chapter 3 explains the processes of choosing and changing your supervisor. This chapter looks at the relationship more deeply and explores what the student should expect from their supervisor, the types of supervisory relationships and some troubleshooting tips for getting the best out of the supervisory arrangements. When you enter a relationship with a supervisor, it is natural to feel fairly unclear about the nature of the relationship because it is not something that is mirrored in other types of relationships, say for example that of a boss and employee. Although there are some similarities, the nature of a PhD does not carry the same hierarchical relationship and often the expectations and parameters are blurred. As one contributor admitted:

When I began to work with my supervisor I had no idea what I could or could not expect of him. He was a very busy head of department and I did not want to make too many calls on his time, but on the other hand I felt very raw and rather overwhelmed with the size and length of the research undertaking. I was not sure I had actually ever done any research before, and I certainly had no idea how I was going to work on a project which would be so lengthy in terms of words and years. [Gina Wisker]

Immediately in the relationship there is tension, expectation, dependency and concern about the huge task ahead. Because of the unfamiliarity of the relationship, it needs to be approached head on and managed constructively from the outset. Your supervisor may well set out clear expectations from the beginning, but if this does not happen then there are some requests you can make and certain actions to take to make sure that you are using the relationship to its fullest capacity.

Types of supervision

It is important to recognise right from the beginning that there are established templates for supervisory arrangements, different forms of supervision and also different styles of supervision. Although 'style', like fashion, is a personal thing, there is something useful to be said about the generic methods of supervision that you may find yourself involved with. First, we will start by acknowledging how supervisors are monitored and checked to demonstrate that there has been increasing emphasis on universities providing good quality and effective supervision.

A safe pair of hands?

The supervisory relationship has been one area that has been dragged into the limelight and bureaucratised in recent years. The Metcalfe Report (2002) examined many aspects of postgraduate experience and reported back to the Higher Education funding councils with the objective of improving standards in postgraduate research programmes. This report introduced a framework of standards and a code of practice for universities to follow in order to protect students and provide effective supervisory arrangements. As a result, supervisory arrangements are now much more institutionalised and go through checks and monitoring processes to ensure quality. Each institution will have its own guidelines about who qualifies to be nominated a supervisor, and the amount and type of supervision that PhD students should receive. For instance, at the University of Leeds the guidelines are for students to receive ten sessions each year. Funders will also want to know who the supervisors are, what experience they have and what the arrangements are for supervisory meetings. Those who have not supervised before will often be mentored by experienced supervisors such as the postgraduate tutor. In addition, there is plenty of guidance and training for supervisors. Departments and universities are also monitored by external quality review processes that examine what is happening at different levels.

The standard code of practice introduced as a recommendation from the Metcalfe Report states that there should be the following:

- A formal agreement between the student and the university.
- Teaching of a series of generic skills.
- A student-held log which records research supervisions.
- Agreed action plans and courses.

Supervisory arrangements are taken seriously by institutions and 'best practice' is expected at all levels. Good supervision can happen in many different forms. Below we look at the three standard types: single, joint and team supervision.

Single supervision

Traditionally, PhDs were supervised by one academic who was considered to be the expert in the subject. This traditional method of just one academic bearing the responsibility for all aspects of the supervision has faded with recent improvements and standards. Perhaps due to the isolated nature of a one-to-one supervisory system, most institutions now offer joint supervision. Nevertheless, whatever form of supervision you are offered, there are some basic requirements of all supervisors. Hockey (1994: 186) summarises that supervisors should:

- Be effective in their organisation and planning with students.
- Communicate with clarity.
- Be flexible and sensitive to student needs.
- Set clear expectations.
- Provide professional guidance.

Joint supervision

The Metcalfe Report recommended that institutions take on a joint supervisory style as part of the framework for standards. They recommended that students have two supervisors to ensure 'increased visibility of the relationship which will give added protection to students' (2002: 22). The sensitive nature of the student–supervisor relationship means that having two supervisors should prevent any major issues arising, and ensure that at least one supervisor is available all year round. Within this dyad, one academic normally takes the lead as the 'main' supervisor. This is often divided based on expertise. Having two people, often with different specialisms and experience, can be refreshing as you benefit from the strengths of each supervisor. For instance, one may be able to advise more on the academic content of the research, while the other could be more tuned to the process of getting the PhD done. Or one may be more methodologically skilled whilst the other is more of an expert in your topic area.

BOX 15.1

Keep records of all your supervisory meetings and important emails from your department and supervisor, and all correspondence with funders. Learn good record keeping.

Team supervision

You may find yourself doing a PhD as part of a larger research team. In this sense you may have one person who takes the lead role, but have supervision with different seniors at different times and for different things! For instance, you could see one person about methodology, another about the management of the actual project and another about academic and intellectual issues. Somewhere in this complex set of relationships you will have to find a way of getting emotional support through what we have been describing as a 'journey'. One of the contributors, Ruth Bartlett, was on a case studentship and part of a larger team working on dementia research:

> A strategy I used to manage what I recognised to be a shift in my working identity was to seek emotional support from an academic supervisor. Because my PhD was a case studentship on a specialist topic I had three supervisors, one of whom was a clinical psychologist. In the early stages of the study I used my sessions with this supervisor to discuss dilemmas I was having, especially about feeling quite powerless.

Even if you are not in a team supervisory situation, you may still choose to use your supervisory arrangements to receive certain types of support and then other mentoring or peer relationships for emotional feedback.

Styles of supervision

The theorising around 'how to be a good supervisor' has started to take off, with books such as *Supervising the PhD: A Guide to Success* (Delamont et al., 1998) acting as bibles for the new, inexperienced and novice supervisor. To summarise issues of supervisor styles, there seems to be two defaults that are in operation when supervisors set out on the rocky path of nurturing students through the doctorate process. These defaults stem from the supervisors' own experiences. Like parents learn to parent from their parents, supervisors often learn to supervise from their own supervisors. Or not, as the case may be. The point is that reflexivity is often an inbuilt process when supervisors develop their own system and methods of communication. These two defaults manifest as follows.

Supervise as supervised

Those supervisors who had a 'good' experience will tend to mirror the supervision they had. For instance, the boundaries or informality surrounding the relationship are usually learned from being supervised; likewise, how to develop effective relationships and create an efficient and safe learning environment are all implicitly learned from 'good' supervision. Often those supervisors who have had good supervision will be clear about the different aspects of the supervisory role and try to 'perform' on all of these.

Supervise as was not supervised

Let's at once dispel the myth that only those who have gone on to work in academia are the products of fine supervision. There will be as many cases of poor supervision as good supervision that academics will have gone through and will use to inform their own roles. This pretty much follows the line, whereby you make a vow that you will not let the same mistakes happen again and set out to 'do things differently'. The learning curve could be more about the interpersonal skills and respect that should be paramount in an effective relationship. No doubt if your supervisor is one who went through hell and back you will find out exactly what the story is.

The ebb and flow of the journey

Your supervisory arrangements will most probably change with the flow of the PhD process. For instance, you are more likely to see your supervisor(s) more frequently in the first year when you are working hard to figure out the research questions, design a feasible project and pass through the upgrade process after the first year. The upgrade process involves preparing a set of documents that are presented to a panel, then, in a viva style interview, you will be asked questions about the project to see if it will meet the criteria needed for a PhD and that you can also do what you are proposing. During this process you will probably see your supervisors more to ensure the upgrade is successful. The year that is designated to fieldwork is often a time when the student is away from the university 'in the field'; this could mean immersed in a situation that is local, or could indeed mean international research. Either way, this year perhaps receives a little less attention from the supervisor as it is trusted that you are clearer on the objectives of the research. The final year of analysis and writing up re-focuses the student–supervisor relationship as the task in hand is to write something useful, critical and analytical. The to-ing and fro-ing of chapter-by-chapter intensifies the relationship, especially in the closing stages of edits and re-writes. At this time you would expect to have more frequent contact with your supervisor.

Overall expectations

We have established that there are different forms of supervision and academics will adopt their own style. But there are some consistent good practices to look out for, and also to act upon if this is not what you are experiencing. It is important to get the outline, objective and purpose of the supervisory meetings clear from the beginning. Gina Wisker recounts how she set up her initial sessions with her supervisor. Doing the PhD part-time and living away from the university meant that there were other issues to contend with as well as working out what the supervisions were for:

> I was a part-time student teaching full-time, living away from the university (120 miles) and commuting to work in another town. We decided after our initial conversations that the best way to proceed would be if he made some suggestions about work to do, I would then read, research, write, extend what he had suggested or cut back as it developed, and as I started to write (he was adamant I should do this immediately so he could learn to work on my writing) to send him some writing in whatever state it was in. I learned to write drafts and phone him up or write and agree a date to send them and to come up and see him.

Gina's account of basing the supervisory meetings around a set piece of work follows a fairly standard pattern. The 'hook' for the meetings is usually written work, but towards the fieldwork stage there can be other tasks such as interview schedules, consent forms, transcripts, sampling frames, coding etc. The thought of having to produce written work from day 1 can seem daunting when you are very much at the beginning of the process. You may feel unconfident about your writing capabilities (this is normal), or not really know what is meant by 'writing a chapter', 'doing a mapping exercise' or 'literature review' (see Chapter 6). But, as Claire Maxwell outlines, positive feedback can be gained from this process, which can help you develop essential skills:

> Getting confirmation from my supervisor that my written work was at a high enough standard to pass for a PhD was crucial in increasing my confidence that I was operating at the right level – something I had really struggled with and doubted.

Setting out work expectations, communication expectations and general ground rules for engagement is a must early on in the working relationship (see Chapter 3). Delamont et al. (1998: 23) set out guidelines for a good relationship with a supervisor highlighting some basic issues, such as choose a 'best time of day' to have meetings, always set an agenda, review the meetings at the annual cycle and respect mutual availability.

Overall, you can expect a range of direct feedback, intellectual discussion, motivation and support from your supervisor. Phillips and Pugh (2005: 147) summarise what students should expect:

- Written work to be read in advance.
- Constructive criticism.
- Good knowledge of the research area.
- An exchange of ideas.
- Supervisor to act as a role model.
- Supervisor to teach the skill of research.
- Short-term goal setting that feeds into longer-term objectives.
- Healthy and helpful 'psychological contract'.

BOX 15.2

Be prepared for a range of criticism: good and bad feedback is the only way to learn and see your work improve.

We would add some additional roles that you can expect from the supervisor:

- Guidance through the fieldwork stage.
- Facilitating access as much as possible.
- Practical advice on 'how to'.
- Giving judgement.
- Advice on careers and steps towards careers.
- Facilitating networking.
- Confidence building.
- Interest in personal development.
- Aware of isolation.
- Enforcing rules and regulations.
- Ensuring you are meeting the deadlines and milestones.

These bullet points are all well and good sitting on this page, but in the real world it must be remembered that academics have their own self-interests when they take on postgraduates. For the supervisor, taking on students can initially be a burden: it isn't clear if the student will work hard and progress at the necessary rate or leave half-way through because the task was too onerous. Be aware that supervisors have their own agenda. Having doctorate students looks good on their CV, provides an opportunity to coach a new researcher and provides a supply of teaching support or research assistants.

In addition, academics are most keen to invest time in students who are interested in similar ideas, willing to take the topic further and be at the cutting edge. Remember, academics do not become supervisors out of the goodness of their heart. Yet remember that students have more to lose than their supervisor if they don't succeed. Box 15.3 provides an example of how one university perceives the supervisor's responsibilites.

BOX 15.3   A research student supervisor's responsibilities include:

- The supervisor will give guidance on research topic, methods, techniques, approach, planning, literature and progress.
- The supervisor should arrange training on subject-specific and generic skills, as well as actively introducing the student to other workers in the field, encouraging participation in conferences/forums/academic societies.
- The supervisor should possess sufficient knowledge of the research area to provide accurate advice and guidance on the project.
- The supervisor must ensure that regular supervisory sessions take place, uninterrupted as far as possible by other business. Both student and supervisor should have a clear, agreed understanding of the frequency and nature of contact required.
- The supervisor should have sufficient available time to dedicate to supervision.
- The student and supervisor must have an agreed procedure for dealing with urgent problems and conflicts. The student and supervisor are encouraged to produce a learning agreement.
- The supervisor should read and provide constructive criticism for all the written work submitted and advise on publications.

(source: http://www.city.ac.uk/researchstudies/rdcforms.htm)

Managing your supervision

The relationship is a two-way street. You will only get out of the relationship what you put in and this means that you need to recognise your own responsibilities in fulfilling your end of the bargain.

Your responsibility is:

- To keep in contact with your supervisor – they will not chase you.
- Supervisors are busy so you need to be at the front of the queue. Always set and keep meetings.
- Be flexible with your times – your supervisor is busier than you are.
- Be honest when negotiating workload – if your supervisor's requests are too much then speak up.
- Once the supervisions are over, if you are not clear, make contact to clarify.
- Make sure you do the work set otherwise inform your supervisor beforehand.
- Do not sit in the dark for several weeks – pick up the phone, send an email, visit during the open door times.

Time is a major factor in all aspects of doing a PhD and time is also an important feature in your relationship with your supervisor. Making sure you see each other at the appropriate time, that each session allows for enough concentrated time (i.e. answering the phone or door is avoided), and that meetings are spaced so adequate time is given in between meetings. Gina Wisker notes how time was a pressure, and she was mindful of the lack of time of her supervisor:

> He and I were both gradually aware of how to enable me to handle the time pressures of research and writing and to manage the different time pressures of my workloads, while I learned not to make enormous or any sudden and unreasonable demands on his time because he was also pressurised, but we did have quality time every time we met and discussed serious issues, and the written work.

Therefore, using both your time and your supervisor's time wisely is essential. Here are some tips on how to use supervisions effectively.

BOX 15.4   Using a supervision session effectively

Before you go to supervisions:

- Constructively plan what you want to accomplish by the end.
- Prioritise your issues.
- Do not use the session just to moan.
- Set out specific questions or an agenda to frame the meeting (these can be emailed before the meeting).
- Make sure no one gets sidetracked and that you get answers.

After supervision sessions:

- If you have missed out questions then email afterwards.
- If there is something you are unclear about then follow up.
- If you have not arranged a date for the next session then suggest one.
- Make sure you are clear about what you need to do before the next session.

Taking ownership of the process

It has already been noted in Chapter 3 that there can be problems in the supervisor relationship: 'The supervisory relationship can be a very private one. In the majority of cases this is an extremely constructive and fruitful partnership, but there are times when relationships break down with consequences for the student, the supervisor and the research' (Metcalfe Report, 2002: 22). Gina Wisker warns that there are several potential misunderstandings about the level of the work, ways of working together, culture clashes and learning styles clashes. This can often manifest when you and your supervisor have different ideas about the direction that your work should take. For instance, it is common for supervisors to have strong feelings about using certain methodological traditions which may not be quite what you had in mind. Or it may be that your supervisor wants you to concentrate on a particular variable and your interests are in other directions. In this instance, the clash is not futile, terminal or insurmountable but just a taster of the academic world where people disagree and have different opinions. The solution does not have to be you giving in to your supervisor's wishes but instead taking ownership of the situation, rationally considering the alternative options and presenting a case as to why your idea should override that of the supervisor. The key thing to remember is that if you have a methodological, pragmatic or theoretical justification for going ahead as you see fit, then this argument should hold weight with your supervisor and in a viva further down the line when you need to explain your actions. At the end of the day it is your PhD, and taking ownership, stating your case and putting your ideas forward can be a liberating experience.

Key Points to Remember

▶ It is a two-way relationship, which means you also have responsibilities.
▶ Learn to approach supervisions professionally.
▶ Plan an agenda for each supervision.
▶ Keep a record of your communication with your supervisor.
▶ You will have limited time from your supervisor, so use it wisely.
▶ Time will be the most important asset.
▶ There are many sources of advice if you think your supervisions are not working. Seek out the postgraduate tutor.

SUGGESTED READING

Eley, A.R. and Jennings, R. (2005) *Effective Postgraduate Supervision. Improving the Student/Supervisor Relationship.* Maidenhead: Open University Press.
Phillips, E. and Pugh, D. (2005) *How to Get a PhD*, 4th edn. Maidenhead: Open University Press.
Wisker, G. (2005) *The Good Supervisor.* Basingstoke: Palgrave.

Chapter 16
Enabling Research Environments

What this Chapter Includes:

▶ Challenging exploitation and enabling student development
▶ Research students and institutional responsibilities
▶ Equal opportunities in the PhD context
▶ Student experiences and institutional practices
▶ Supervision and additional part-time academic work
▶ Enabling access to facilities, resources and equal opportunity
▶ Knowing your rights as a research student

Challenging exploitation and enabling student development

This chapter considers universities as institutions with responsibilities to provide a safe, supportive and enabling learning and research environment. We also acknowledge the persistence of some exploitative and discriminatory practices within doctoral student experiences (see below Graves and Varma, 1997; Hockey, 1994; Phillips and Pugh, 2005). There has been a concerted effort within universities to improve standards across institutions and realise equality of opportunity for access to Higher Education. The Dearing Report (1997) provided a major impetus for revising the standards of the PhD research programme, and particularly the supervisor–student relationship. The Higher Education Funding Council for England (HEFCE) supported a revision of standards of the Code of Practice in academic quality set out by the Quality Assurance Agency (2004). For doctoral students, this meant the academic appeals process and student complaints procedure was strengthened and the general monitoring and support for PhD students was standardised. We hope to enhance student awareness of the statutory and ethical duties of universities in order to help protect against and address unsatisfactory practices – many of which are the result of unintentional actions and embedded cultures. As we shall see, there are aspects to the research student–supervisor–institution relationship that can encompass grey areas. The PhD can be viewed as an 'academic apprenticeship' but can also involve 'exploitation' if additional paid work opportunities leave the research student unprepared or underpaid. Likewise, the significance of 'autonomous study' or 'independent learning' can be hampered if underpinned by elements of supervisory or institutional neglect. These issues can be complex to judge owing to highly subjective perspectives and are rarely appropriate topics for discussion within departmental activities. While research students have ultimate responsibility for their research, and to actively seek and utilise the resources and facilities within your own institution and those available to the academic community, universities also have increased responsibilities through regulation and equal opportunities legislation formalising more aspects of the research student–university relationship.

In this chapter we will consider common vulnerabilities research students can experience, such as feeling unable to refuse unpaid or ill-conceived research or teaching assistant work. Additionally, some particular students have been recognised as needing more targeted support, such as disabled students, in order to access post-graduate research opportunities. Raising awareness of your own and the university's rights and responsibilities will be important to enhance your awareness. With these concerns in mind, the chapter begins with a brief overview of the institutional framework of support for PhD students in the UK, with a discussion of recognised good practice. We then turn to consider some student experiences in relation to the supervisor–student relationship, taking on additional academic-related work during your PhD and seeking support for particular needs such as those related to having a disability or being a student with caring responsibilities. The final section of the chapter reviews the varied nature of institutional and personal practices, reflecting on some of the points raised in the first section when thinking about ways of negotiating an enabling research environment that suits your professional and personal development needs.

Research students and institutional responsibilities

The framework of legal and institutional regulations and services surrounding post-graduate research and learning has changed considerably in the past few years within UK universities. There has been a concerted effort to enhance the quality of provision and teaching, so that universities and key personnel – such as supervisors, Boards of Studies, postgraduate tutors, human resources, student support services and heads of department – have a clearer and regulated role in respect to research students. Legislation relating to equal opportunities in a more general sense and specific changes to doctoral supervision aim to set out the rights and responsibilities of research students, supervisors, other department personnel and other university services, such as student support services for disabled students. The support needs of international students, students who are parents or carers and disabled students, have become more widely recognised as well as the need to address exploitative and discriminatory practices and cultures.

Equal opportunities

If you seek out your university's equal opportunities and anti–discrimination policies and codes of practice (accessible via the human resources/personnel department web page or main contacts), you will hopefully find that something similar to the following mission and principles inform them:

> This university is committed to equal opportunities in all its activities. It is intended that all students should receive equal treatment irrespective of political belief, gender, sexual orientation, age, disability, marital status, race, nationality, ethnic origin, religion or social background. (City University, London, July 2006)

The drive to establish equal opportunities within Higher Education in practice, however, continues to be a challenge as the changes required involve attitudinal, cultural and institutional change. Further objectives, such as widening participation agendas, need to be balanced against meeting institutional targets in other areas. Universities seek to extend the diversity of their student cohort and adapt their educational practices in order to fulfil widening participation objectives. The quote from City University below demonstrates the kind of cultural and institutional changes and vision required. Equal Opportunities is not merely about dismantling direct and indirect discrimination – it is about realising the contribution a diverse cohort can make to an institution and providing equal opportunities as a principle of social justice and rights rather than privilege:

> City University believes in the principles of social justice, acknowledges that discrimination affects people in complex ways and is committed to challenge all forms of inequality. To this end, City University will aim to ensure that:

- individuals are treated fairly, with dignity and respect regardless of their age, marital status, disability, race, faith, gender, language, social/ economical background or being lesbian or gay and any other inappropriate distinction;
- it affords all individuals, students and employees the opportunity to fulfil their potential;
- it promotes an inclusive and supportive environment for staff, students and visitors;
- it recognises the varied contributions to the achievement of the University's mission made by individuals from diverse backgrounds and with a wide range of experiences. (City of London, Equal Opportunities Policy 2006)

Equal opportunities policies and legislation, therefore, are in place to promote equality of opportunity within a university, to promote good working relationships between students and staff and to address unlawful discrimination. As a research student, and member of the university community, you have a right to equality of opportunity and treatment in ways that contribute to your well-being and development. For your own awareness or in the event of feeling you have a grievance to address, seek out your institutional policies in this area. Box 16.1 provides a guide to the kind of support and key personnel to find out about.

Student experiences and institutional practices

Supervision and additional part-time work

While it is important to resist the 'I blame my supervisor for all my PhD problems' mantra and recognise the two-way responsibilities and challenges that the supervisor–student relationship entails, research students can become prey to exploitative practices, which in many cases can be quite unintentional, arising from the culture of an organisation or assumptions about the supervision process. There is an inherent power and authority imbalance within student–supervisor relationships as students are far more dependent on their supervisors than the supervisors are on research students. Research students rely heavily on their supervisors as a source of research and wider academic advice and support. A good supervisor who is knowledgeable in your research area, aware of their responsibilities and seeking to enhance your academic career can not only impart very important academic and research advice, but can also help you to access professional contacts, dissemination opportunities and even future academic jobs. Within this relationship, however, raising concerns about your supervisors' performance or not taking forward their advice can be a tricky situation to navigate. Added to this is the possibility of non-compatibility due to differences in learning and teaching expectations and preferences. As we stated in Chapters 3 and 15, you will need actively to manage this relationship in order to negotiate the supervisory support conducive to your learning style and needs.

An example of the complexity of these issues is offered from our anonymous contributor below:

Soon into my studentship, I started working part-time on a voluntary project, which was set up by my supervisor. I felt it was a big opportunity and could not believe I had been asked to do such a job! I felt lucky at getting such good experience. However, it was not made clear to me at the beginning, the extent of the work. I was dealing with a lot of press inquiries and the job gradually took over from my PhD research, especially once the main project worker left and I ended up more or less running the project.
[Anonymous]

After getting little done on her PhD in her second year, our contributor started to raise concerns about her research progress and the overwhelming nature of the voluntary project role. However, with her supervisor expressing confidence in her ability to get her PhD done alongside her other role our contributor thought her own concerns about her PhD progress were unfounded. It was only later on, after a year or so reflecting on this stage in her PhD, that our contributor felt her concerns were not listened to or recognised by her supervisor. Our contributor gradually felt more and more detached and de-motivated as a research student.

Feeling indebted to your supervisor for wider academic opportunities can be common among research students. Our contributor in this case felt in hindsight she had over-valued this wider experience, and with little progress on her PhD she decided to take a year out from her studies and began working full-time at the university in a teaching capacity. The final outcome was that she did not return to her PhD study and even gave up her new employment as she became 'exhausted' and ill.

There is a silver lining to this cloud, however, as we met our anonymous contributor when she had returned to start afresh on a new doctoral project at a different university, where she felt happy with her supervision and more focused on her PhD research.

The issues this example raises are interesting. It is common for research students to value the opportunity to take on additional academic work for their supervisor. It can feel flattering that your supervisor values your competence to the point of offering you such opportunities. But opportunities can turn into risks and exploitation – especially in terms of the time, effort and resources that are required, and the degree to which the work complements your doctoral project. We would recommend that you carefully consider any such work and allow for frequent reviews of how such work is progressing your research and your career. A guide for good postgraduate working opportunities is available via the links referenced at the end of this chapter.

Enabling access to resources and opportunities

Universities can vary quite considerably in the facilities and resources offered to doctoral students but the minimum facilities and resources should include a desk, computer, library access and supervision. Our contributors below, who are both disabled students, provided examples of how the support available had to be actively sought and the additional effort this required:

> When I tried to register in my first week I soon discovered that registration was being held in a huge hall only accessible by an old stone staircase. I had to ask a fellow new-comer to register for me! If I had known this situation in advance I could have made alternative arrangements. Universities are getting much better at supporting disabled students but that support also has to be actively sought after. In my early days information from the university disability support services was vague and always needed to be followed up for clarity.
> [Rebecca Mallett]

Rebecca felt emotionally drained and quite isolated from her experiences of needing to plan her studies and activities quite carefully to accommodate her physical impairment and the barriers to opportunities that other students could take for granted:

> It's draining and laborious to be the only one thinking through how other people's decisions (e.g. which room to book for a seminar) might affect your ability to participate. When doing fieldwork with an impairment you often feel uncertain, vulnerable and quite helpless at times. I often vented frustration in my research journals and there are many extracts in them discussing how, during fieldwork, I was unable to make the detailed plans I normally did because I had to rely on so many things and so many other people.

Another PhD student, Sonali Shah, felt it took her a while to find out about her rights to support, while she was coping with feeling quite isolated owing to her physical restrictions that meant she could only study at her computer in her bed-sit and not the shared postgraduate study area:

> On such occasions I felt very isolated. This isolation was also due to the fact that I was working from my student bed-sit and had very little social contact with other PhD students who worked together in a research room. One of the primary reasons

I worked alone and not in the research room was the fact I needed specialist IT support, which was set up on my personal computer but not on any computer in the research room. I now realise I should have not let this happen. I should have been much firmer about my rights and the support I required – and asked for this IT to be available elsewhere. I felt the disability advice service did not provide much support or advice for me as a postgraduate.

Universities can offer disabled students help with specialist accommodation, software, personal assistants and equipment – but what is offered also needs to not lead to isolation. Finding and negotiating this additional support takes time and effort:

The effects of my physical impairment prevented me from completing and submitting my PhD within three years, which fitted the university and funding timetable. Doctoral research took me longer as I also had to rely on personal assistants, who are not experienced researchers, to locate relevant publications for me, time that is not accounted for in the official time allocated to complete a PhD. Furthermore, the turnover of personal assistants during my studies was high. Therefore significant time was taken up advertising for and training new personal assistants to assist me. Having to rely on personal assistants also influenced my fieldwork in terms of when I could conduct the interviews.
[Sonali Shah]

In this instance, Sonali was able to gain a further year as her supervisor approached her funder directly and effectively negotiated an extension. Rebecca felt more positive about the institutional support for disabled students:

I am fortunate to be funded by a research council, have access to a 'non-medical helper' fund through DSA (Disabled Student's Allowance) and have a brilliant disability adviser. She acts as a liaison between me and my department and the research council. Through DSA I employ support workers to help me access places that are inaccessible, such as the library building.

Again, the emphasis may be on you to be informed of your rights to support. Additional support can also be available in terms of academic language support for students' for whom English is a second language and for students with children.

Knowing your rights as a research student

It is possible, therefore, to set out some guiding principles and a vision of student rights. A major problem for research students can be the isolating effects of working on an independent piece of work that takes several years to complete – increasing your dependence on your supervisory support. However, you should not suffer alone if you feel your institution is not providing the support and guidance you require. Dealing with any problem as quickly and as early as possible will help things not to escalate and threaten your progress. Primarily, thinking through the nature of your problem and concerns, getting them formulated in your own thoughts and raising them with your supervisor or an alternative trusted staff member in an informal capacity are important first steps. Secondly, finding out about your institution's policies, codes of practice and complaints procedures will empower you to act and follow the more formal routes of redress if necessary.

In principle, the National Union of Students proposes that students have the right to the following ten conditions – and that these conditions also enable equality of opportunity within Higher Education. In particular, we would like to highlight the rights listed under numbers 3 to 10 as crucial to enabling opportunity for a diverse research student cohort.

BOX 16.2   The NUS student bill of rights

The NUS believes every student has:

1   The right of access to post-16 education and a fair financial system of support
2   The right to representation
3   The right to study free from discrimination, prejudice and fear
4   The right to adequate support facilities and learning resources
5   The right to clear and accessible complaints and appeals procedures
6   The right to safe, secure and affordable accommodation
7   The right to a fair and equitable wage for safe part-time work
8   The right to suitable childcare provision
9   The right to be involved in Student Union activities
10   The right to be a citizen of an academic and wider community

---

Overall, a central message of this book is to propose a proactive and informed student approach. Therefore, you also have the right to find out and get to know exactly what is expected of you when you embark on your doctorate–academically and financially; and to negotiate an enabling learning environment that provides a balance between your own responsibilities for your studies and those of the university.

Key Points to Remember

▶ Universities are regulated by equal opportunities and quality assurance legalisation aimed at addressing discrimination, enhancing teaching and student support.

▶ Get to know the key personnel within your university, department and academic community who have a role in supporting doctoral students.

▶ Think about your rights as a student to an enabling learning environment and opportunities – do not suffer in silence if you are concerned about the standard of supervision or support you are receiving.

▶ Research students can be particularly vulnerable to poor supervision, informal or low-paid part-time working conditions and isolation.

▶ There is additional support provision for disabled students, international students and students with children, but this support will probably have to be actively accessed by the student.

▶ Find out about organisations that support student welfare – such as the National Postgraduate Committee (www.npc.org.uk).

SUGGESTED READING AND RESOURCES

Graves, N. and Varma, V. (1997) *Working for a Doctorate*. London: Routledge.

Hockey, J. (1994) 'New territories: problems of adjusting to the first year of a social science PhD', *Studies in Higher Education*, 19, (2): 177–190.

National Postgraduate Committee (1992) *Guidelines on Codes of Practice for Postgraduate Research*. Available at www.npc.org.uk/thenpc/npcpublications

National Postgraduate Committee (2005) *Guidelines on the Provision of Exclusive Postgraduate Facilities*. Available at www.npc.org.uk/thenpc/npcpublications

Phillips, E.M. and Pugh, D.S. (2005) *How to Get a PhD*. Maidenhead: Open University. Ch. 9 and 12.

Chapter 17

Combining Family Commitments and Doctoral Studies

What this Chapter Includes:

▶ Balancing multiple roles, identities and responsibilities
▶ Incompatible and competing roles and identities
▶ Personal and academic belonging
▶ Complementary and empowering connections
▶ Postgraduate students with children
▶ Strategies for success

Balancing multiple roles and responsibilities

Over the course of this book we have illustrated how undertaking a doctorate is a huge commitment that is rarely taken lightly. It is an endeavour that will take at least three years to complete. Over that time, you will be undertaking an academic and a personal journey of change and development. In this chapter we look at the experiences of, and issues raised by, students undertaking a doctorate while also having family responsibilities. The discussion also has a wider application if we consider the inter-connections between our personal lives and academic lives. Our lives and aspirations rarely fit into neat and distinct categories as students, employees and so on. Rather, students negotiate expectations and activities relevant to being a research student alongside expectations and aspirations for their own well-being and as partners, family, employees and community members (also see Chapters 11–14 in Part III of this book for consideration of combining employment with doctoral studies, the 'personal' nature of the doctoral journey and non-traditional routes into the PhD; also see Chapters 16 and 18 on aspects of personal well-being and welfare).

In this chapter we cover four key aspects of combining family responsibilities and doctoral studies – competing roles and responsibilities, complementary connections, institutional support and developing your own strategies for success. Within these areas we cover issues such as seeking childcare, accommodation, financial support and other resources and services as well as experiences of and strategies for overcoming, the sometimes conflicting nature of academic and family roles along with recognition of complimentary connections.

Incompatible identities, roles and responsibilities?

Juggling multiple responsibilities and demands

Combining raising children with doctoral studies can feel like an impossible juggle between multiple expectations and demands (including those we place on ourselves and those imposed on us by others). Much will depend on the extent of your caring responsibilities, the size of your family, the age of your children, health needs, income levels and partner/social network support. It is common for student surveys to report some degree of incompatibility while juggling family responsibilities and doctoral studies (Edwards, 1993). You may feel anxious about or actually overstretched by the demands on you and unsure if family, fellow employees and friends understand the significance that your doctoral research holds for you and the commitment it entails. Partners, friends or dependants may at times also express concerns about feeling 'second place' to your PhD!

A complex set of personal, cultural, financial and institutional factors shape parental experiences and much can be done in our view to help students cope and reduce such conflicts. Our contributors indicated concern about the impact of doctoral study on family life as well as that of family life on doctoral study. While undertaking doctoral research is rarely a straightforward decision for any student, students with family responsibilities often have to weigh up the costs and benefits for their family as a whole, especially if the family income may be reduced, or whether everyone will be willing to uproot to live nearer the host university. David felt undertaking a PhD could be a 'risk' for his family. David began doctoral study after several years in full-time language teaching employment. Taking up a PhD studentship meant a considerable reduction in the family income and change in the family 'lifestyle':

> When considering doing a PhD after a career I had to weigh up the pros and cons of leaving work to become a student again and was faced with a number of difficult questions. You can be filled with apprehension and self-doubt: 'I haven't written or read anything academic for years!' 'Am I too old to be a student?' 'Surely everyone on the course will be used to studying and I'll be the "odd one out"?' 'What will my colleagues, friends, and family think if I leave a job to become a student again?' Take financial matters – unless you are in the enviable position of knowing now that you are realistically able to finance three or four years of PhD study – there are a number of difficult financial matters to consider (this is all the more so given the fact that, as a mature student, it is probably more likely that you will be faced throughout your studies with having to meet ongoing financial commitments which younger, 'pre-career' students are less likely to be faced with, such as a mortgage, bills, and children). This will call for meticulous (and, if you have a family, *collective*) financial planning.
> [David Smith]

Edwards (1993) refers to the anxieties mothers can feel in undertaking projects that indicate self-aspiration rather than service and care for other family members. David above indicated the 'risky' decision for many in taking a reduced salary in order to follow a doctoral programme. While we hope undertaking a PhD will be beneficial for your family as a whole, and an endeavour supported by your family and friends, this may not always be the case. Strain can appear, such as when you need concentrated time alone to study, think and write, or when you are struggling with a period of uncertainty about the direction or conclusions of your research. These times can be very all-consuming and individual in nature.

When contemplating PhD study later in life, the compatibility of PhD study with 'life as you knew it' before is an issue. I found there was a massive shift from a lifestyle that revolves around a career and 'regular' family living patterns to the lifestyle of a PhD student. The scale of these changes should not be under-estimated, and anyone contemplating a PhD will have to consider the extent to which family and friends will be supportive of the new direction your life has taken, as well as the extent to which you will be able to shape your family life around the needs of PhD study. PhD 'working habits' can be highly irregular, and often come in short bursts of hectic activity in which you find yourself deeply engaged in late-night reading and writing sessions, followed by moments of relative calm, where deadlines have been met, write-ups completed, conferences attended, interviews completed, etc. Further, PhD study often leaves you with a sense of isolation as well as a need for individual study, of being locked away from the world with 'your' project which nobody else understands or is particularly interested in.
[David Smith]

In a survey posted on a UK university postgraduate forum, one mature student vividly paints a picture of juggling competing demands, with a 'resolution' involving working at home as much as possible, which was also problematic as this led to isolation:

Like any working mother I am constantly juggling. At first I struggled to come to meetings and courses that clashed at every point with child care and parent care and part-time work commitments and social life. The latter is not a luxury but an absolute necessity if you are working largely on your own. Early evening courses might fit in with part-time studying but not if you have children as well. I attempted to make contact with other students. I failed. I managed to continue by basing myself at home and working from there as I used to do as a freelancer. I came in for supervision and for necessary meetings. (Liesbeth de Block, Learning Matters   k1.ioe.ac.uk/learningmatters/studforum.htm)

Negotiating time and space for your doctoral research within your family routine and environment can be challenging, and may require much flexibility, negotiation and explaining on everyone's part. It is fairly unrealistic to think you can leave your thoughts on your PhD at the door on coming home, or that you can leave your personal family issues at home when you go to university. Thinking about how your PhD and family life will impact on each other will be helpful for you to identify such strains and talking through mutual expectations and demands is recommended by some students:

> You will need to ask yourself how PhD demands might affect family commitments. Will you be able to integrate these rather unstable demands into family life, and will family members be able to accommodate the sudden changes and new element of unpredictability which doing a PhD entails? Will you be able to negotiate a 'space' for your studies – a place exclusively for your desk, books, papers, computer and notes, where you are guaranteed time to maintain the intense degree of concentration which your studies will demand? Will you face severe restrictions in your study times and working habits (students with fewer family/home commitments, for example, may like to work late at night rather than throughout the day – an option which is not open to everyone).
> [David Smith]

Dislocation and difference: bridging family and academic belonging

Although there are more undergraduate and postgraduate students with children today compared to ten or twenty years ago, there can still be a popular image of the traditional student being one who is younger and without caring responsibilities. Additionally, many supervisors can expect long hours of studying as evidence of doctoral commitment – and studying for a doctorate will necessitate much individual study in practice. Whether a fiction of our insecurities or a dominant cultural imaginary – research students with children can feel different compared to images of the mainstream student. Anxieties around 'fitting in' can be particularly overwhelming and can be real barriers to participating in group social activities or academic seminars/conferences, especially if these are within out-of-school hours. Mature students can feel less familiar with conventions of oral or written academic communication but becoming conversant in academic disciplinary discourse is a must for success (Wisker, 2001).

On the other hand, research into the experiences of non-traditional students, especially those who are parents, older or from more minority ethnic or working class backgrounds, has noted how research students find that their research interests and work become incomprehensible to their families (Morley, 1999). However, this situation can lessen over time as families and friends themselves become more conversant with your academic role, and personal well-being can be enhanced by actively seeking and building support networks with other mature students with family responsibilities.

It is also worth thinking through your preconceptions. Harriet Churchill felt that she had 'internalised a position of disadvantage and anxiety' in the early stages of embarking on doctoral research. She was surprised to meet other doctoral students with family responsibilities:

> I was concerned about how I was going to balance looking after my pre-school child with doing my studies. Having looked after my daughter full-time for two years I was unsure how she would take to full-time nursery. I was also worried about whether I would be able to join in on out-of-nursery-hours events and seminars. However, to my surprise another first year research student had a young child, which challenged my preconceptions of being so different.

Research students with family responsibilities can also experience very real constraints in accessing and completing doctoral research. Our contributors and our research have particularly noted time, finances, accommodation and childcare constraints as key issues. Students with family commitments report feeling time-stretched, with a daily trade-off between attending a networking event, meeting fellow students for lunch or getting your head down to study when you only have school hours and evenings for research! This adds to the strain of wondering whether you are 'doing enough' and 'being productive'. Immersion in study sometimes has to be organised around the routines set for children, sometimes leading to studying late into the night or before the children rise the next day. At times students who are parents feel excluded from evening seminar or social events. However, Harriet felt that whilst being a mother with a young child did restrict her autonomy as a doctoral student it also provided a clear boundary between her doctoral activities and the rest of her life:

> I felt very 'time pressured' – constantly aware of time – time I had spent studying, time I had taken out. Once my daughter was attending school (the nursery hours fitted better with full-time working hours) my day at university was structured by the school day, which ends at 3pm. My studying day at the university felt shorter than many of my fellow PhD students. I attempted to 'catch up' with my studies by studying until late into the night after children's bedtime! In hindsight I am not sure how productive this strategy was as then I was tired the following days. However, motherhood was also my area of research so my experiences were a rich source of critical inquiry for me. Further, being a mother and having a caring role for a young child was also an alternative set of commitments and very consuming, so that I was able to switch off from my studies.

Complementary and empowering connections

Harriet makes a significant point about the empowering and complementary nature of combining family responsibilities with doctoral research, which we would also like to recognise and encourage students to think about. Above, Harriet describes her appreciation of having clear 'boundaries' in some senses – such as those relating to a daily structure between 'family time and PhD time', so that family responsibilities offered an alternative role and time out from thinking about and doing doctoral-related work. Alternative viewpoints have moved beyond a purely 'constraint or limitation' perception of family responsibilities in relation to doctoral research. Not only do parents bring valuable skills and attributes to their studies and university activities, such as organisational, communication and adaptability skills, they also bring a wealth of life experience. Further, their children are likely to become aware of Higher Education possibilities and activities. If you are concerned about your competence or training needs as a research student, having returned to formal education after many years of absence, do not suffer with these anxieties alone – universities now run many training courses or can help with funding and academic development in a broader sense beyond your specific research training needs. Uncertainty, anxieties and self-doubt if recognised and not pathologised could be thought through in a process of self-reflexivity and identification of what is needed to enhance the doctoral process and offer important learning opportunities for you. This might include seeking additional support, identifying training needs or acquiring a mentor. Indeed, it is in recognition of the need to support PhD students in a more regulated way that many universities now offer annual training needs audits with each student, in line with quality assurance recommendations.

Institutional support for postgraduate students with children

Within your institution, there may be access to provision and support for childcare, your own and your child's welfare, accommodation, flexible access to research student facilities and resources, financial support and informal peer support. There are also a number of government departments and advice organisations that can offer help with visas, additional financial support and childcare advice for students. The National Union of Students has also published guidelines for good practice (see below), which can provide a checklist against which to find out about provision and support within your university or indeed can be a yardstick to campaign for better provision.

Access to affordable and accessible childcare is crucial in enabling many people to undertake doctoral research. For Harriet Churchill the institutional policy and provision for childcare was favourable:

Particular good aspects of the university nursery provision were income-related fees, a free settling in period before my studies commenced and the on-campus location. For me as a PhD student the fees were at the lowest rate, which all students paid, which was about half the average local rate for full-time nursery childcare at that time. There was an on-site nursery only a few minutes' walk away from the departmental offices. With the ability to relocate a couple of months before the beginning of my PhD, there was also the advantage of the nursery policy to gradually build up towards full-time attendance over a few weeks, thus potentially easing the transition for child and parent.

The National Union of Students (see nus.org.uk) campaign for four key aspects of good practice in institutional provision of childcare for students and staff stipulates:

1   Childcare arrangements must be flexible to suit the needs of students with children of various ages within and out of school hours and terms.
2   As a supplement to this, bursaries for child-minding should be available for students for whom home-based childcare is appropriate.
3   The student should be given sufficient flexibility to be able to cope with emergencies if they arise. This applies to attending meetings and seminars, amongst other areas.
4   Institutional environments must be safe for students to bring their children. If this is not possible (e.g. in the case of laboratories) there should be an area where children may be safely left alone for a short period of time.

Another important source of information is childlink.gov.uk, which is a national website that advertises childcare providers on a locality basis and provides advice and guidance for parents seeking childcare. There are some good examples and practice guidelines on childminding contracts and list of questions to ask prospective providers.

Advice, counselling and information

Your Students' Union Advice and Welfare Centre, Graduate Student Support Centre or Accommodation Office should also be able to assist you with advice on visas, employment rights and taxation and welfare benefit issues. Another valuable service that can be available is counselling, offered to students on a one–off basis or as a longer-term arrangement. Counselling may help in thinking through any difficulties you are experiencing in your academic or personal relationships and activities (see Chapter 18).

Other key organisations will be the National Union of Students (NUS), National Council for One Parent Families, National Institute for Family and Parenting,

Parentline, and the Department for Education and Skills (DfES, contact details in Suggested Reading below). Contact your local Social Services Department if you feel you need a Carers Assessment – by law Social Services are required to carry out such an assessment if you are caring for a relative. They take into account your status as a student and the needs of the carer/cared-for. They can offer respite or home help services.

Financial support and accommodation

It is worth inquiring about family-orientated university accommodation as this can be cheaper than alternative accommodation for families and centrally located near the university. Research students on studentships funded by research councils or universities are also eligible for top-up Access to Learning funds, which are also available for low income UK students who are deemed in need of extra financial support. It is worth investigating the application procedure and eligibility via your student welfare advice service. Students with children (especially lone parents), students with partial or no funding and disabled students are particularly targeted. Students on low incomes may also be eligible for Working Tax Credit and Child Tax Credit.

There are also a number of trusts and charitable organisations that seek to assist low income or disadvantaged postgraduates, often for specific activities such as conference attendance or publications. Details of these organisations are available via the Trust/Charity Guide, which is annually updated and available within most public and university libraries.

Strategies for success

Finding a balance between your family and research responsibilities and activities will enhance your well-being. While your university and other organisations may be able to help you with access to support, flexibility with deadlines if needed, and financial assistance, students themselves are adept at generating coping strategies. Our contributors particularly valued making time and taking the effort to build up an informal social network (see Chapter 18). Talking through problems with family, friends and supervisors at the earliest possible stage was also advised as a good way of preventing a larger problem in the end. Recognising you are on your own academic and personal journey may also be an important viewpoint to consider. Comparing yourself to senior academics (who may be your age) or fellow PhD students with no caring responsibilities beyond themselves and friends, may not be a matter of comparing like with like. Such comparisons can lead to dents in your self-confidence. Recognise your achievements and personal learning, indeed celebrate and reward yourself for reaching minor and major milestones. We advocate auditing and taking action on your organisational, research, basic literacy and technical skills – your PhD can be a time of personal development in a variety of ways (see Chapters 14 and 18 in particular).

▶ Students negotiate expectations and activities relevant to being a research student alongside expectations and aspirations for their own well-being and as partners, family, employees and community members.

▶ Embarking on and getting through doctoral research while having family responsibilities can involve conflict and tensions, such as multiple expectations on your time, attention and resources.

▶ Mature students returning to postgraduate study after some years out of formal education can feel concerned about their academic competences, the impact on family life of becoming a student and fitting in with the wider academic community.

▶ Times and locations for seminar and social activities can conflict with family demands.

▶ However, support is available via your university Student Welfare Service and Students Union.

▶ Other organisations and government agencies can also help students with financial support, information for childcare provision and help with accommodation/research costs.

SUGGESTED READING AND RESOURCES

Department for Education and Skills (2006) *Childcare Grant and Other Financial Support to Full-Time Students Who Are Parents*. Available at www.dfes.gov.uk/studentsupport/uploads/ChildcareGrant0506.pdf

Simon, L. (2005*) New Beginnings: A Reference Guide for Adult Learners*. Hemel Hempstead: Prentice-Hall.

Chapter 18

Coping with Stress

With Eve Parsons, Practising University Counsellor

What this Chapter Includes:

- ▶ An account of the stresses and anxieties that naturally occur as part of undertaking a PhD
- ▶ A review of the place of counselling in the Higher Education sector
- ▶ Recognition that PhDs are taken within the context of other life issues
- ▶ How issues with your supervisor can be dealt with
- ▶ Why counselling may be needed at different stages of the PhD
- ▶ How to address procrastination
- ▶ Reflections from a practising counsellor about what university counselling may offer

The stresses and strains of the birth of a thesis

By now this book should have convinced you that taking on a PhD is an exercise in emotional and intellectual stamina that is more like an extreme rollercoaster ride than a pleasant walk in the park. The level of personal commitment needed in order to succeed is very difficult to express in words as it is like an intangible energy that propels you forward to the end. What is easier to convey is that at some point along the line you may well need additional support from your supervisor, and/or family and friendship networks to deal with the very normal stresses and strains of this intellectual and emotional journey. Nearly all students go through various stages of angst, insecurity, confusion, isolation and depression at some point. Kurtz-Costes et al. (2006: 137) note that doctoral students feel the pressure from frequent evaluation, financial duress, competitive atmosphere, low status and high workload. All these anxieties are often based on a complex relationship between the personal journey of doing the PhD, the difficult intellectual task and dealing with the external outside world which has no real idea what a PhD is!

Do not feel as if you have failed, or that your coping strategies are substandard: the fact is that doing a PhD is difficult and manoeuvring over and around the emotional and psychological pitfalls is part of the task. Many of the negative feelings and phases you will experience can be buffered by your personal and academic support networks. For instance, a good old moan to a fellow comrade in the pub, a series of focused meetings with your supervisor, a holiday (yes – you are allowed to take time off) or getting further immersed in networking or fieldwork can shift the problem. But there may be times when you feel that you do not want continually to burden your partner or friends with the stress of your day job, or you may get fed up with your mother offering tea and sympathy and feel that an independent and objective ear would be more helpful.

Sniffing out support

The university counselling services, available in the majority of institutions, may be able to offer guidance and solutions to your anxieties. The good news is that these services are offered free of charge at the point of access by most institutions. The difficult bit is plucking up the courage to go and seek help, admit that the problem is one that you cannot solve on your own, or even open up about your innermost fears to a stranger.

BOX 18.1

Find out what support services your institution provides for postgraduates, such as student advice services, financial advice services and a confidential counselling service.

The PhD process requires an immense intellectual depth that is usually correctly assessed at the time of being offered a place to study for a doctorate. In most cases, the intellectual ability needed to succeed is not what is in question, but problems can arise when the emotional skills and capacity that are required to go through this intellectual task are not as robust as they need to be. What is often forgotten by the outside world is that a doctorate is not really like a job that has a 9–5 structure, or can be easily switched off in the evenings or during vacations. This is why when other life stresses are apparent, the PhD candidate may experience issues differently from someone who is in a regular, mainstream occupation.

Early on, as much as is possible, learn to protect your social and personal time and space from the demands of your PhD. Try to keep up a balance by remaining involved in other activities such as sport or hobbies, even if this is at a reduced frequency.

In situations where the normal routes of support such as family and friends or spending more time with your supervisor do not prevail, specialist help may be needed. The university setting provides various points of help, such as the Student Union and the university's own student support services. Both of these provide paid staff who can assist with university systems and protocols such as requests for temporary suspension of registration, and complaints procedures. In addition, there are mainstream support services in the local town/city that can be accessed, through self-referral or via your GP, irrespective of your postgraduate status. Nevertheless, there may also be times during the PhD process when you feel that problems are arising or escalating and that a different kind of assistance is required.

The role of the counsellor

Counsellors are usually employed by the university and so they have a specific contract with the institution in the same way that the student is also part of the institution. The services provided are normally on a one-to-one basis for short- or longer-term contracts, with group counselling sessions as an alternative. Some institutions offer group work specifically for postgraduates. To reflect the structure of the PhD, counselling is often available throughout the year, including vacations, recognising that PhDs don't stop during the summer months!

The fact that the service is 'internal' may be a point of anxiety for students who query issues of confidentiality and what is actually going to happen to the information imparted. This is a particular issue when the problem is about the supervisor! Yet, be assured, university counselling services work within a strong commitment to maintaining confidentiality and abide by a set of ethics that honours and protects the student's wishes not to have information revealed to other persons in the university. Bound by the confidentiality codes set out by professional bodies (such as the British Association for Counselling and Psychotherapy and the UK Council for Psychotherapy), confidentiality is breached only in rare and extreme circumstances (and this is most likely to be to a doctor). Counsellors always seek to discuss widening confidentiality with their clients if at all possible before doing so. Information is only shared with academic departments with the consent of the student.

Counselling provided within the Higher Education setting has the particular benefit of being geared to the student experience, especially the somewhat strange (and strained) lifestyle of the doctoral student. Counsellors in the university setting are well aware of the lifestyle of a student, who is embroiled in different types of relationships and protocols, that carry power dynamics perpetuated by the embedded hierarchies (for instance, based on class, gender and ethnicity) that Higher Education is traditionally built around. Higher Education is a peculiar setting, with intense relationships with peers and supervisors which are not often mimicked in other areas of life. Recognising these as common problems that are specific to the student experience is half the solution.

Counselling provides a safe space to explore your feelings and difficulties with a view to finding your own solutions. In addition, with your consent, counsellors can sometimes (depending on the service's policies) provide relevant evidence if you want to request special arrangements over deadlines or negotiate time-out from studies. In this respect, the counsellor can take on a more significant role in terms of practically supporting the doctoral student to balance coping with the demands of personal problems alongside those of the PhD in difficult times.

Likely issues – more than a blocked sink

A lot of the issues that counsellors deal with are about personal lives; whether it is a current relationship breakdown, for example, or experiences in the past that have come to the fore and need to be dealt with. But equally it is the process of the PhD and the isolation that often accompanies being a doctoral student that are familiar reasons for visiting a counsellor, frequently because the student is experiencing anxiety or depression. Points of tension can also be the relationship with the supervisor, relations with peers and how PhD students establish themselves in their department.

The normal external pressures and everyday life events do not go away or become less significant just because an original piece of academic work is under way. The Royal College of Psychiatrists (2003) recently alerted medical services to the extent of mental health problems amongst students in HE. This was associated with the significant stress factors of making so many transitions at once. Any stressful life event (bereavement, relationship breakdown, physical illness, unexpected pregnancy and so on) can throw the PhD off track. Or overseas students, who may have made considerable personal sacrifices (i.e. leaving family behind) to study in the UK, may experience a 'cultural disjunction' between home and their temporary residence (see McNamara and Harris, 1997). In addition, deeper more long-standing issues may also come to the surface for the first time – especially if these are entangled with the research topic. Problems can re-surface – something that was sorted un-sorts itself owing to the stress of the PhD. Let's not forget that the traditional age bracket for doing a PhD is between 22 and 30, which is a stage of life when one is establishing oneself as an independent adult. At this stage, identities are often in flux, making the journey of a PhD possibly more stressful. Sexuality and relationships are often highlighted in this stage anyway, but coupled with the new experiences that the PhD process brings, a student can often feel overwhelmed.

BOX 18.4

Doing a PhD can provoke emotional states that may increase your anxieties. Unblocking your personal issues is often the only way to move the PhD forward.

Many of these types of problems that are unearthed as a result of studying take years to sort through. Sometimes students do not feel they have the luxury of time to deal with life issues during the PhD because of the pressure of the three-year deadline. Unfortunately, emotional healing cannot be fast-tracked and often compartmentalisation can be an alternative solution by putting a lid on the issues while work goes on. Counsellors can support students who choose this coping strategy too.

Financial pressures are never far away from the constant niggles of the postgraduate lifestyle. Even with studentships and teaching opportunities, money is always tight, with increasing rents and books to buy. Often part-time jobs are a solution to the financial difficulties but taking on additional work can also increase the pressure of having less time to study. Financial pressures are not only current but also cumulative, as often by this stage you have been a student for a number of years, and with tuition fees, the student debt mounts up. Even though repayment can normally be suspended during postgraduate study, debts are always looming in the background, waiting to pounce once a decent salary starts flowing into the current account.

Another issue that is often discussed with a counsellor is that of your changing role and the conflicts this brings. As a doctoral student you have to make a significant shift from the role of the undergraduate, and this can bring with it confusions in itself. Hockey (1994), in a study titled *The Social Organisation of Postgraduate Training,* reported that at the beginning of a PhD research students struggle with the change in status. Hockey also highlights that 'the problem which students face is that their new position is ambiguous, in as much as it is at best only vaguely defined by university regulations'.

The conflict around status can also be related to taking on a new teaching role. Taking on an additional pastoral and teaching role brings responsibilities and stress, especially if teaching is new. This is a particular concern for those students who have teaching bursaries and are expected to take on a significant amount of teaching and marking but at the same time to get their project off the ground. Whether your undergraduate years were two or ten years ago, there is always some kind of role change taking place. You may have been a full-time parent or a manager of a company before you embarked on a PhD. Whatever your change in status, this can bring with it specific anxieties, so don't be too harsh on yourself.

BOX 18.5

If you are an older student, remember that all PhD candidates are going through some kind of role and status change (see Chapters 11 and 17).

Isolation is one of the central problems experienced by doctoral students. The feeling of having a mountainous task and no one really understanding what this actually entails is part of the course. Surrounding yourself with people who are in the same boat is essential, especially for those who are registered part-time. Community building is initiated in the first year through courses about the PhD process and other opportunities that encourage communication through peer presentations and support groups. A range of introductory talks that may seem trivial (the library tour for instance!) actually enable other essential types of networking. After the first year, students tend to be geographically spread out because fieldwork kicks in and people disperse into various fieldwork sites in other localities. So peer groups have their own ebb and flow as people come and go, making loneliness a likely friend. Again – this is not just happening to you, so seek out others to share what's going on.

The wrath of the supervisor

As a doctoral student you will find your morale and sense of well-being are affected by your supervisor(s) which in turn influences motivation and focus. As highlighted in Chapters 3 and 15, establishing an adult relationship – which does not deal only with the business side of the task but is a holistic working partnership – is the key to a successful mentoring relationship. The list of potential problems that can arise is endless, but some of the common pitfalls that can be the reason for seeking counselling are changes in supervisors, people being away and unavailable, serious issues such as unfair treatment in terms of (for example) racism and sexism, and feeling inadequately supported. As many universities favour the joint supervision approach, difficulties can arise for students who are left trying to balance contrasting views of two or three supervisors. Fathoming out whose advice is best and trying to meet even some of their requirements without treading on toes can become stressful.

Relationships of power are endemic in the student–supervisor interaction. Often the supervisor is a senior member of the academy – perhaps someone whom you have admired through reading their work and listening to them speak for some years. This kind of relationship can initially be frozen; you feel you are working with someone so eminent, or just someone who is so good at their job, that your abilities seem trivial and inadequate. Such intimidation can usually be managed where there is friendliness, but where there are issues of approachability or transparency (when you really don't know what your supervisor should be doing for you), monthly supervisions can be terrifying! The flipside to this is that you may have a very approachable (often younger) supervisor who regularly takes you for coffee and asks about your dog but is not an expert in your field of study and therefore your confidence wanes in their ability to give advice. With younger supervisors their lack of experience may also trouble you in terms of their authority, knowledge and track record of getting students to the end. Sometimes there are others in the department who can offer advice (for instance the postgraduate tutor), but these stresses can leave scars that may need attention.

BOX 18.6

Be clear from the start with your supervisor about your and their expectations and the format of the supervision sessions. This sets up boundaries and a precedent early on (see Chapter 3).

Even when there are no obvious problems with the supervisor, just negotiating this new type of relationship that is integral to your experience and work is a strange phenomenon. When rapport is not instantaneous, or the relationship feels far too much like that of a parent with their child, then there may be perceptions and concerns to unpick. The relationship between the supervisor and PhD student has new parameters and boundaries that must be negotiated and understood – often implicitly. The relationship is often at odds with that which you have experienced as an undergraduate, where the role was very functional and based on seniority. There is a different kind of relationship at the postgraduate level – one where the supervisor may assume a more pastoral role. This relationship is more of a 'horizontal' relationship where more intimate knowledge about each other's personal life is shared and the spaces that the relationship is conducted in move beyond the department to the pub! This adult-to-adult relationship, where informal socialising is often an important part, complicates boundaries and in some cases closeness can become a problem as it transgresses expected boundaries.

Stages of stress

When considering the stresses associated with the PhD, it is worth realising that problems can arise at different points. You may have sailed through the first year, collected amazing original data and then hit a sticky point – or indeed the test of character could have come in those initial months. Either way, there are some key triggers when the PhD process can falter, leaving you stuck in the mud. The beginning and the end appear to be points when students often require additional support. The foundation year makes a difference to the rest of the experience, so a shaky start could leave insecurities. Feeling behind already or realising you are not as suited to the PhD process as you imagined, can make the second year feel like it will go on forever. However, additional support, including counselling, is often most needed during the writing up phase, when there can be both physical and psychological manifestations of stress. Running out of editing time, or even ideas, putting in monotonous hours in front of the computer, or requiring extra support from a 'time-short' supervisor can all become too much. At all of these stages, what Hockey (1994: 182) has termed 'a struggle with intellectual self-worth' can become the sticking point as we develop a lack of confidence in our 'intellectual selves'. Additional support may be useful to talk all this through.

Procrastination

The PhD process has inbuilt mechanisms to ensure that procrastination (the avoidance of doing a task) does not set in or that writer's block does not spoil the whole enterprise. Formal upgrades, progress reports and regular meetings with supervisors, which include deadlines for short pieces of work, generally map the development of the PhD. However, from interviews with PhD students, Hockey (1994: 181) concludes that 'time becomes a source of anxiety' for the lone scholar. Students are told from the outset that the expected completion time is three years. When time is pressured so that we feel like 'every hour counts', then stagnation for even a week can seem like a long-term procrastination problem. This may not necessarily mean that professional help is needed at this stage but if you feel the problem persists then this is something that perhaps can be addressed through cognitive behavioural strategies – making simple changes to your thinking and behaviour that can have positive effects. However, with procrastination also come feelings of guilt, failure, inadequacy and letting others down. These negative feelings can lead to problems such as depression. Be aware of these potentially damaging effects of negative feelings about the self and remember there are various sources of help.

BOX 18.7

Always have some administrative tasks to do if writer's block sets in. Useful tasks include: sorting out the bibliography, scanning tables of contents of electronic journals, browsing the library, writing your CV, reading a decent newspaper, writing an abstract for a conference.

Do not think, however, that all of the issues mentioned above need long-term intervention to help you find solutions. You may find it only takes a couple of hours talking to someone impartial about what's on your mind to help you find a balance.

No magic wands but …

Counselling is a broad umbrella term for a process that can offer the following aspects:

- A safe, confidential space to off-load.
- Space to explore feelings and choices of action.
- Re-framing the problem away from blaming yourself to more constructive thought patterns.
- Dealing with expectations that are out of proportion.
- Learning to be self-aware.
- Learning to be assertive.
- Adopting new emotional skills and emotional literacy.
- Accessing other support services within and outside the university.
- Liaison with supervisors and departments informally and sometimes formally.
- Time management, stress management and self-care.
- Group work to share issues and combat isolation.
- Cognitive behavioural strategies to tackle personal and social anxieties.

Bear in mind that:

- Many institutions only have a small team of counsellors, so there may be a waiting list to get seen on an ongoing basis.
- The counselling provided may only be over a short time period, although there might be the opportunity to re-access the service later.

BOX 18.8

Lots of people have counselling – it doesn't mean something is wrong with you!

Key Points to Remember

- ▶ All students go through some wobbly stages when the emotional and intellectual strain takes its toll. This is not failure, but part of the process.
- ▶ Life doesn't stop and PhDs are not done in a bubble. Other life events may need addressing through one-to-one support.

▶ Specific stresses relating to the PhD are isolation, relationships with supervisors, time and financial pressures, role and status change and procrastination.

▶ Use your friendship and personal networks alongside your academic sources of support to gain various insights and some perspective on what may seem like insurmountable hurdles.

▶ Most institutions offer a specific student counselling service that is free at the point of access.

▶ Counsellors work under strict codes of confidentiality and normally information is not shared with others unless with your consent.

SUGGESTED READING AND RESOURCES

Hockey, J. (1994) 'New territory: problems of adjusting to the first year of a social science PhD', *Studies in Higher Education*, 19 (2): 177–190.

McNamara, D. and Harris, E. (1997) *Overseas Students in Higher Education: Issues in Teaching and Learning.* London: Routledge.

Perry, A. (2002) *Isn't It About Time? How to Overcome Procrastination and Get On with Your Life.* London: Worth.

www.studentcounselling.co.uk
Guide to problems and solutions
FAQs for students

Final Thoughts

Having made your way through the many aspects of the PhD we have outlined in this book, we want to provide you with some final words of reassurance and suppress any anxieties that may have been raised about the enormity of the task ahead. These final thoughts are offered in the spirit of wishing you every possible success and strength for the wonderful journey of gaining the PhD.

Dispelling the myths

What we have tried to do in this book is to dispel some of the lingering myths about what doing a PhD means, who normally enrols as a PhD research student and the process of gaining a doctorate. We hope to have taken you through the pitfalls of getting the right supervisor and maintaining good working relationships. We have provided tips on how to think coherently about your research questions; presenting your work; how to avoid missing the deadline; and to remember that there are safeguards and flexibility that you can call on in times of need. Doing a PhD is hard work and personal circumstances will, in some cases, make the process of doctoral study more challenging. But be assured, the traditional 'type' of student who moves from undergraduate to postgraduate status within Higher Education in their early 20s is a rare breed these days. Diversity amongst postgraduates is increasingly the norm. We feel that there can only be strength in a wide and varied research student base, from which everyone can give and take support and build those important networks.

Designing your personal strategy

Throughout the chapters, the summary boxes have provided a range of advice, anecdotes, strategies and further points of information to help you to build your own personalised strategy to successfully tackle the hurdles of the PhD. By now you will have a clear idea of how some of these issues are likely to be raised during your journey. You will know where your weak points are, be aware of where to seek out support, what your rights are as a student and your entitlements. We hope we have stirred some capacity to be proactive about getting what you want at every level. We have dedicated two chapters to the role of the supervisor in the PhD process, which suggests the importance of this relationship. However, although we have emphasised this as crucial to your smooth passage through the system, we also want to stress that it is not uncommon for these relationships not to work out. So when they don't, please don't personalise this too much. Rather, seek out help and find someone more suitable. Having the correct supervisor and the right sort of supervision is not the only way to gain support. This is why we have highlighted the importance of networking and attending postgraduate and discipline-specific events.

Isolation is a significant part of doing a PhD because of the autonomous nature of the job and the fact that the ultimate responsibility for the whole project comes down to you. Your personal strategy must include mechanisms to deal with this. While we have given you plenty of tips on how to design a strategy for your three years, please also take ideas from our diverse contributors because there is no one set way of proceeding. Successful strategies can come in many shapes and forms.

The personal and professional journey

We are particularly proud that this book tackles something close to both our own experiences and beliefs: that the PhD is a personal as well as a professional journey. We have been keen to include and combine the importance of considering the personal as well as the professional when designing your own strategies for success at every stage of the process. At the beginning, having frank discussions with yourself and your loved ones about what taking on a PhD means will be important because everyone will have to make sacrifices. Your own personal circumstances that lead you to enter Higher Education will dictate why you are embarking on this solitary task and what hurdles may lie ahead. But embrace these challenges as part of the process and rather than see them as hurdles allow them to be opportunities and chances to learn more about yourself and your research. This is where 'reflexivity' really comes into play, as you will find taking stock important in research as well as in your personal life.

Remember to have fun!

We have deliberately taken a generally serious tone in this book because of the weightiness of doing a PhD, the scale of the effort required and the fact that some people never finish because of the difficulties. Yet, here we want to remind you that, as we can testify, doing a PhD will be an enjoyable experience and very likely a life-changing one. It is a time for growth, experimentation, newness, socialising, travel and fun. Don't be afraid to enjoy! This is the flipside of the sacrifices and compromises you and others will have to make, so when opportunities come by to lighten the load, do take them. The art of effective time management is being able to have it all!

Stepping stones

Despite the seriousness of undertaking a doctorate, we do not want you to leave this book thinking a PhD has to be a masterpiece and therefore might be unachievable. We offer you this little snapshot from one of our contributors, who sums up how the PhD should be put into perspective:

> About a month before I was due to start my doctorate, a colleague and mentor turned to me as we were about to cross the road near Trafalgar Square and said 'Do your best, enjoy the experience, but remember it isn't going to be a masterpiece, its just your first step onto the academic career ladder'.
> [Justin Waring]

If you are not intending to stay in academia, then the stepping stone principle still applies. Getting a PhD is just one of the milestones along the personal and professional journey.

After writing this book, if we were asked to consolidate some general advice for postgraduate students, we would not re-invent what has been said before but instead refer you to Les Back (2002). His top ten hints (he calls them aphorisms) for getting through your PhD are:

1 Trust your own interest
2 Keep a ledger of your thinking
3 Read promiscuously with an open mind
4 Don't become addicted to the library
5 Don't be afraid to get close to the thing you're trying to understand
6 Don't become a fieldwork junkie
7 Embrace the challenge of becoming a writer
8 Don't carry the burden of originality
9 Don't try to judge your own work
10 Have faith in the value of what you are doing

These are useful nuggets of advice to follow and incorporate into your own personal strategy. Finally, remember where you are heading and, in those times when you want to pack it all in, remember:

> By completing our studies, our intellectual skills become honed and nurtured; our research techniques, whether empirical or theoretical, are developed and proven; our managerial, administrative and teaching abilities are enhanced; and our findings and ideas are worked-up to a standard that awards a doctorate. We therefore have much to offer.
> [Justin Waring]

References

Arksey, H. and Knight, P. (1999) *Interviewing for Social Scientists*. London: Sage.

Arnold, J. (1997) *Managing Careers into the 21st Century*. London: Paul Chapman.

Atkinson, P., Coffey, A., Delamont, S., Lofland, J. and Lofland, L. (2001) *Handbook of Ethnography*. London: Sage.

Back, L. (2002) 'Dancing and wrestling with scholarship: Things to do and things to avoid in a PhD career', *Sociological Research Online*, 7 (4) at www.sociologicalonline.org.uk/7/4/back.html

Back, L. (2004) 'Ivory Towers? The academy and racism', in I. Law, D. Phillips and L. Turney (eds), *Institutional Racism in Higher Education*. Stoke-on-Trent: Trentham Books. pp. 1–6.

Becher, T., Henkel, M. and Kogan, M. (1994) *Graduate Education in Britain*. London: Jessica Kingsley.

Becker, L. (2004) *How to Manage Your Postgraduate Course*. Basingstoke: Palgrave.

Blaikie, N. (2000) *Designing Social Research: The Logic of Anticipation*. Malden: Polity Press.

Blaikie, N. (2003) *Analysing Quantitative Data*. London: Sage.

Boice, R. (1994) *How Writers Journey to Comfort and Fluency: A Psychological Adventure*. London: Praeger.

Bourner, T., Bowden, R. and Laing, S. (2001) 'Professional doctorates in England', *Studies in Higher Education*, 26(1): 65–83.

Britton, C. and Baxter, A. (1999) Becoming a Mature Student: Gendered Narratives of the self. *Gender and Education*, 11(2): 179–193.

Collinson, J. (2003) 'Working at a marginal "career": the case of UK social science contract researchers', *Sociological Review*, 51(3): 405–422.

Coomber, R. (2002) 'Signing your life away? Why Research Ethics Committees (REC) shouldn't always require written confirmation that participants in research have been informed of the aims of study and their rights – the case of criminal populations', *Sociological Research Online*, 7(1) at www.socresonline. org.uk/7/1/coomber.html

Crang, M. and Cook, I. (2006) *Doing Ethnographies*. London: Sage.

Crow, G., Wiles, R., Heath, S. and Charles, V. (2006) 'Research ethics and data quality: the implications of informed consent', *International Journal of Social Research Methodology*, 9(2): 83–95.

Curnock, A. (1996) *Quantitative Methods in Business*. Cheltenham: Stanley Thornes.

Dearing Report (1997) Higher Education in the Learning Society. Available at www.ncl.ac.uk/niche/sr_008.htm

Delamont, S., Atkinson, S. and Parry, O. (1998) *Supervising the PhD: A Guide to Success*, 2nd edn, Buckingham: Open University Press.

Department for Education and Skills (2003) *The Future of Higher Education*. London: HMSO.

Edwards, R. (1993) *Mature Women Students*. London: Taylor and Francis.

Elbow, P. (1973) *Writing Without Teachers*. Oxford: Oxford University Press.

Employed Postgraduates' Charter (2003) www.npc.org.uk/page/1050329840

Finch, J. (2003) 'Foreword: Why be interested in women's position in academe?', *Gender, Work and Organization*, 10(2): 133–136.

Gibbs, G. and Coffey, M. (2004) 'The impact of training of university teachers on their teaching skills, their approach to teaching and the approach to learning of their students', *Active Learning in Higher Education*, 5(1): 87–100.

Graves, N. and Varma, V. (1997) *Working for a Doctorate: A Guide for the Humanities and Social Sciences*. Routledge: London.

Harland, T. and Plangger, G. (2004) 'The postgraduate chameleon', *Active Learning in Higher Education*, 5(1): 73–86.

Hartley, J. and Fox, C. (2004) 'Assessing the mock viva: the experiences of British doctoral students', *Studies in Higher Education*, 29(6): 727–738.

Higher Education Statistics Agency (2005) Online Information Service, Student Data Tables. www.hesa.ac.uk/holisdocs

Hockey, J. (1994) 'New territory: problems of adjusting to the first year of a social science PhD', *Studies in Higher Education*, 19(2): 177–190.

Holt, S. (1999) *Preparing Postgraduates to Teach in Higher Education*. Coventry: Council for Graduate Education.

Howard, K., Sharp, J.A. and Peters, J. (eds) (2002) *The Management of a Student Research Project*. Aldershot: Gower Publishing.

Jackson, C. and Tinkler, P. (2001) 'Back to basics: a consideration of the purposes of the PhD viva', *Assessment and Evaluation in Higher Education*, 26(4): 355–366.

Joint Statement of the UK Research Councils? Training Requirements for Research Students, (2001) The UK grad programme, www.grad.ac.uk

Kurtz-Costes, B., Andrews Helmke, L. and Ulku-Steiner, B. (2006) 'Gender and doctoral studies: the perceptions of PhD students in an American university', *Gender and Education*, 18(2): 137–155.

Le Voi, M. (2002) 'Responsibilities, rights and ethics', in S. Potter (ed.), *Doing Postgraduate Research*. London: Open University and Sage. pp. 153–163.

Lee-Treweek, G. and Linkogle, S. (2000) *Danger in the Field: Risk and Ethics in Social Research*. London: Routledge.

Leonard, D. (2001) *A Woman's Guide to Doctoral Studies*. Buckingham: Open University Press.

Lester, S. (2004) 'Conceptualizing the practitioner doctorate', *Studies in Higher Education*, 29(6): 757–770.

Letherby, G. (2003) *Feminist Research in Theory and Practice*. Maidenhead: Open University Press.

Marks, A. (2003) 'Welcome to the new ambivalence: reflections on the historical and current cultural antagonism between the working class and higher education', *British Journal of Sociology of Education*, 24(1): 83–93.

Mason, J. (2002) *Qualitative Researching*, 2nd edn. London: Sage.

McNamara, D. and Harris, R. (1997) *Overseas Students in Higher Education: Issues in Teaching and Learning*. London: Routledge.

Metcalfe Report (2002) www.hefce.ac.uk/pubs/hefce

Miller, T. and Bell, L. (2002) 'Consenting to what? Issues of access, gate-keeping and "Informed" consent', in M. Mauthner, M. Birch, J. Jessop and T. Miller (eds), *Ethics in Qualitative Research*. London: Sage.

Morley, L. (1999) *Organising Feminisms: The Micro-Politics of the Academy*. New York: St Martin's Press.

Morss, K. and Murray, R. (2005) *Teaching at University: A Guide for Postgraduates and Research*. London: Sage.

Murray, R. (2002) *How to Write a Thesis*. Maidenhead: Open University Press.

Murray, R. (2003) *How to Survive Your Viva: Defending a Thesis in an Oral Examination*. Maidenhead: Open University Press.

Murray, R. (2004) *Writing for Academic Journals*. Maidenhead: Open University Press.

Osborne, M., Marks, A. and Turner, A. (2004) 'Becoming a mature student: how adult applicants weigh the advantages and disadvantages of Higher Education', *Higher Education*, 48(3): 291–315.

Phillips, E. and Pugh, D. (2005) *How to Get a PhD*, 4th edn. Maidenhead: Open University Press/McGraw-Hill Education.

Punch, K.F. (2000) *Developing Effective Research Proposals*. London: Sage.

Quality Assurance Agency (2004) Code of practice for the Assurance of Academic Quality and Standards in Higher Education. http://www.qaa.ac.uk/academicinfrastructure/codeofpractice/

Raddon, A. (2002) 'Mothers in the academy: positioned and positioning within discourses of the "successful academic" and the "good mother"', *Studies in Higher Education*, 27(3): 387–403.

Rangasamy, J. (2004) 'Understanding institutional racism', in I. Law, D. Phillips and L. Turney (eds), *Institutional Racism in Higher Education*. Stoke-on-Trent: Trentham Books. pp. 27–34.

Ribbens, J. and Edwards, R. (eds) (1998) *Feminist Dilemmas in Qualitative Research*. London: Sage.

Rickards, T. (1992) *How to Win as a Mature Student*, London: Kogan Press.

Roberts Review (2002) *SET for Success: The Supply of People with Science, Technology, Engineering and Mathematical Skills*. Report of Sir Gareth Roberts' Review, 15 April 2002. www.hm-treasury.gov.uk

Robertson, J. and Bond, C. (2001) 'Experiences of the relation between teaching and research: what do academics value?', *Higher Education Research and Development*, 20(1): 5–19.

Rugg, G. and Petre, M. (2004) *The Unwritten Rules of PhD Research*. Maidenhead: Open University Press.

Sanders, T. (2005) 'Researching sex work: dynamics, difficulties and decisions', in D. Hobbs and R. Wright (eds), *A Sage Handbook of Fieldwork*. London: Sage.

Sanders, T. (2006) 'Sexing up the subject: methodological nuances in researching the female sex industry', *Sexualities*, 9(4): 449–468.

Tinkler, P. and Jackson, C. (2004) *The Doctoral Examination Process*. Maidenhead: Open University Press.

UK Grad Programme (2004) *A National Review of Emerging Practice on the Use of Personal Development Planning for Post Graduate Researchers*. www.ukgrad.ac.uk

Wellington, J., Bathmaker, A., Hunt, C., McCulloch, G. and Sikes, P. (2005) *Succeeding with Your Doctorate*. Sage Study Skills. London: Sage.

Wilkinson, D. (2005) *The Essential Guide to Postgraduate Study*. Sage Study Skills. London: Sage.

Wisker, G. (2001) *The Postgraduate Research Handbook*. Basingstoke: Palgrave.

Wright, T. and Cochrane, R. (2000) 'Factors influencing successful submission of PhD theses', *Studies in Higher Education*, 25(2): 181–195.

Example of an Informed Consent Form

My name is Sharon Elley and the purpose of this consent form is to tell you of your rights as a participant in this study and of the procedures involved in the collection and keeping of data about yourself. I am interested in young people's views on sexuality, sex and relationship education, and sexual relationships. I would be very grateful for your participation in this study.

Research and what you need to know

- It is your right not to answer any question that you are asked
- You may ask the researcher any questions you have
- You are free to end your participation in the interview at any time without giving a reason and without any consequences
- Your name and identity will be changed so no one will be able to recognize you in the study and you are guaranteed confidentiality in any discussions and publications in agreement with the Data Protection Act 1998
- No information will be passed onto anyone connected with you, including parents or school
- If you are under 18 and disclose physical, mental or sexual abuse I cannot guarantee confidentiality and this will be passed on to the appropriate persons
- The interview will be recorded using audio tape and all notes and tapes will be kept in a safe place
- You have the right to access the data about yourself and to ask for it to be returned to you at any time

I have read this consent form in full. I have had the chance to ask questions concerning any areas that I did not understand. I consent to being a participant in the study:

    Signature of participant:

    Printed name of participant:

    Date of interview:

    Signature of interviewer:

If you want to confirm that I am a research student at the University of Leeds, Department of Sociology and Social Policy, please contact [my supervisor] on: [phone number]

Appendix 2
Example of an Information Sheet

Young People's Views about Sex and Relationships

I am Sharon Elley and I would like to invite you to take part in some research that is all about **YOU** and **YOUR VIEWS** about sex and relationships in general. **YOUR** opinions are what counts and you receive a £5.00 voucher. It's easy, it only takes about half an hour to an hour and it's up to you.

My research project aims to find out about:

- What sex education you had at school?
- What you learnt from your sex education classes?
- Whether sex education influences what you do?
- What you think about close relationships?

You can help by taking part in this research and telling me your views. You can do this by:

- Taking part in a group discussion with your friends
- Taking part in a discussion on your own with me in privacy

Any information you give me will be strictly confidential. This means:

- None of the information will have your name on it
- No information will be shown to parents or anyone else who knows you
- No one will be able to identify you in anything written

You will not have to answer any questions that you do not want to.
   If you are interested in having your say then please contact me on: [phone number]

If you want to confirm that I am a research student at the University of Leeds, Department of Sociology and Social Policy, please contact [my supervisor] on: [phone number]

Thank you

Index

family commitments *cont.*
  financial support 201
  parental experiences 195–8
female students 131–2
field of study 24
fieldwork
  field notes 62–3
  and part-time study 145
  personal emotions 167–8
  personal safety 55–6
  preliminary 23, 26
finance and funding 6, 17, 191, 201, 207
focal research questions 24
free writing 76

generative writing 76
goal setting 107–9, 110–12, 148
grey literature 88

information sheet 220
informed consent 47–9, 219
institutional responsibilities 185–8
isolation 135, 143–4, 206, 208

job search 122–5
joint supervision 33, 177

learning agreement 182
legislation *see* regulations
life experiences 15–16, 165–7
literature review/overview 24–6, 89
loneliness *see* isolation

management *see* project management;
    time management
ManuScript 88
marking 160–1
mature students *see* older students
mentors *see* supervisors
Metcalfe Report 176
motivation
  core reasons 13–17, 20
  and life experiences 15–16, 165–6
  older students 130–1
  part-time study 141

National Union of Students 192, 200
networking 71–2, 95–104
  anxieties and relationships 96–7, 98–9
  benefits of 95–6, 100
  constraints and commitments 102–3
  isolation/loneliness 135
  non-academic groups 101–2
  part-time study 148–9
  peers and own university 99–100
  and publishing 92–3

networking *cont.*
  research communities 97–9
  seminars, conferences and workshops 100–2
NUD*IST 63–4

older students 129–39
  isolation/loneliness 135
  personal circumstances 131–2, 195,
      196, 197–8
  professional doctorates 137–8
  role and status change 208
  transfer of job skills 132–4
ontology 31
Open University 140, 161
oral examination *see* viva

papers and publishing 71–2, 83–94
  career development 85
  co-authorship 87
  conferences 79–80, 92–3, 101
  content of papers 84
  criticism/peer review 84–5, 88, 90–2
  hierarchy of 87
  publishing process 89–90
  rejection 90–1
  self-confidence 84
  thematic papers 67–8, 78
  timing 83, 85, 86, 88
  what/where to publish 86–8
part-time study 4, 140–9, 165
  coping with isolation 143–4
  distance learning 129, 140, 165
  motivation and preparation 141–2
  prioritisation 146–7
  supervision 180, 188–9
  support and networking 148–9
  time management 144–6, 147–8
peer networking 99
peer review/criticism 84–5, 88, 90–2, 181
perfectionism 108–9
personal agenda 15–16
personal circumstances 102–3,
      109–10, 113
  disabled students 190–2
  family commitments 194–202
  older students 131–2
  part-timers 144, 146–7
Personal Development Planning 7
personal experiences *see* emotions
politics
  and passion in topic choice 19–20
  research as 16
post-graduate training 2–4
  changing framework 4–6
  institutional responsibilities 185–8
  transferable skills 5–6, 132–4